GU01006538

The Gold Standard

The Challenge of Evidence-Bas(
and Standardization in Health Care

The Gold Standard

The Challenge of Evidence-Based Medicine and Standardization in Health Care

STEFAN TIMMERMANS
AND MARC BERG

TEMPLE UNIVERSITY PRESS
Philadelphia

To Lehna and Merel

Temple University Press, Philadelphia 19122
Copyright © 2003 by Temple University
All rights reserved
Published 2003
Printed in the United States of America

♾The paper used in this publication meets the requirements of the American National
Standard for Information Sciences—Permanence of Paper for Printed Library Materials,
ANSI Z39.48-1984

Library of Congress Cataloging-in-Publication Data

Timmermans, Stefan, 1968–
  The gold standard : the challenge of evidence-based medicine and standardization in
health care / Stefan Timmermans and Marc Berg.
    p. cm.
  Includes bibliographical references and index.
  ISBN 1-59213-187-5 (cloth : alk. paper) — ISBN 1-59213-188-3 (pbk. : alk. paper)
  1. Medical care—Standards.   2. Evidence-based medicine.   I. Berg, Marc.   II. Title.
RA399.A1 .T564 2003
362.1'02'18—dc21   2002044388

2   4   6   8   9   7   5   3

Contents

Acknowledgments

THE SEEDS of this book were sown in October 1998, at the Society for Social Studies of Science conference in Halifax, Nova Scotia. Drinking hot chocolate on a patio filled with reminders of the *Titanic*'s demise, we took stock of our research endeavors. We were both involved in a number of discrete projects that dealt with attempts at rendering medical practice more uniform and transparent. From the common and complementary themes that repeatedly emerged in our research projects, it quickly became apparent that if we joined forces our argument would be stronger, and we could aspire to reaching a wider audience. Chapters moved electronically back and forth over the Atlantic Ocean until they gradually lost much of their origins and formed the building blocks of a unique, cohesive argument.

In this book we take a step back from the often heated rhetoric of standardization in health care—critics shudder at the mindless sameness of standards, while supporters dream of a world in which standardized "best practices" orient health care providers—and look at how standards, protocols, and guidelines actually affect health care. Most commentators are aware that standardization is a powerful process. If used well it promises to render medicine more accessible, cost-effective, and democratic, but if used wrongly it is said to stifle creativity and health care delivery into a bureaucratic straitjacket. Our reference point is evidence-based medicine, a strongly backed movement in the contemporary health care field aimed at making recommendations on how to practice medicine to individual health care providers based on a systematic evaluation of scientific evidence. Situating evidence-based medicine historically allows us to explore the politics of standardization via clinical practice guidelines and other standardization tools. From students learning the tricks of the health care trade, to individual health care practitioners providing treatment, to third parties reimbursing and regulating care, we discuss how standardization helps to reconfigure people, instruments, and interventions to foster new notions of autonomy, objectivity, medical jurisdiction, and risk. Cutting through the hype and fears, we study where the potential powers of standards lie. The point of our book is to show how standards are not about less or more skills, or more or less uniformity, but about a redefinition of autonomy of patients, of relationships. In short, standards are about creating new worlds. Not necessarily brave new worlds: the point of this book, ultimately, is to show how many *different* worlds standards can help bring into being.

We have been greatly inspired by the work of Leigh Star, Geof Bowker, Bruno Latour, and Annemarie Mol—distinguished members of the club of people interested in seemingly boring but actually crucially important topics. Leigh and Geof have persistently and kindly shown the importance of looking at standardization from the perspective of those aligned with standards and those left out of the standardization loop. Bruno and Annemarie, in their turn, have opened our eyes to the social life of things, and to the importance of making *differences*. We also thank Olga Amsterdamska, David Armstrong, Ruth Benschop, Wiebe Bijker, Peter Conrad, Antoinette de Bont, Steve Epstein, Mark Elam, Els Goorman, Sarah Lamb, Donald Light, Erica Lundback, Michael Lynch, Agnes Meershoek, Debra Osnowitz, Andy Pickering, Trevor Pinch, RITHM (Marc's research group for Research on IT in Health Care Practice and Management), Laura Neumann, Evelleen Richards, Anneloes van Staa, Irma van der Ploeg, Diane Vaughan, and John Harley Warner for their valuable insights and comments on preliminary versions of this manuscript. Marc thanks Klasien Horstman, Saskia Plass, Paul Harterink, and Michele van Heusden for the joint work on the history of paper records and the study of insurance physicians that was crucial for parts of Chapters 1, 2 and 4. Stefan thanks Alison Angell for conducting research used in Chapter 5, and Valerie Leiter for her collaboration on the thalidomide material. Emilie Gomart has supported us in a myriad of ways—intellectual, gastronomical, emotional, infrastructural—providing us with the generous constraint that pushes one further. Special thanks also to Ruth Baxter who gracefully tolerated, even humored, our talk about these largely invisible tools of medicine.

Some earlier versions of chapters have been published as journal articles. Parts of Chapter 1 have been published in M. Berg and P. Harterink (in press), "Embodying the Patient: Records and Bodies in Early Twentieth Century U.S. Medical Practice," *Body and Society*. Some parts of Chapter 2 have been published in S. Timmermans and M. Berg (1997), "Standardization in Action: Achieving Local Universality through Medical Protocols," *Social Studies of Science* 26 (4): 769–799. An early version of Chapter 4 has been published as M. Berg, K. Horstman, and S. Plass (2000), "Guidelines, Professionals and the Production of Objectivity: Standardization and the Professionalism of Insurance Medicine," *Sociology of Health and Illness* 22: 765–791. An early version of Chapter 5 was published as S. Timmermans and A. Angell (2001), "Evidence-Based Medicine, Clinical Uncertainty, and Learning to Doctor," *Journal of Health and Social Behavior* 42 (4): 342–359. A version of Chapter 6 has been published as S. Timmermans and V. Leiter (2000), "The Redemption of Thalidomide: Standardizing the Risk of Birth Defects," *Social Studies of Science* 30 (1): 41–72.

Back in Nova Scotia while we were contemplating the pros and cons of collaborating on a book, Marc was about to become a parent and Stefan became a father a year later. We dedicate this book to our delightful and mischievous firstborn daughters, Lehna and Merel. While we were immersed in writing, our offspring mastered mobility and language: they learned to scuttle, crawl, stumble, walk, climb, tumble, and run, to coo, mimic, sing, word, name most farm animals, imagine stories, and narrate their adventures. Childhood experts almost unanimously advise that children need structure and rules. Yet, the twinkle in our daughters' eyes when violating a "standardized" rule we had only set ten minutes earlier made us, once again, understand both the importance and the limitations of standardization.

Introduction
The Politics of Standardization

IN 1991, leading international emergency medicine researchers gathered in the beautifully restored, 800-year-old Utstein Abbey on Mösterey, a small island off the southwestern Norwegian coast. In this breathtaking setting of green hills surrounded by wild seas, the international task force engaged in the very basic work of defining what counts as first aid life-saving behavior and how it should be recorded. Since the early 1960s, cardiopulmonary resuscitation (CPR) has been the principal first aid method of reviving victims of sudden death in the Western world. Whenever somebody suddenly collapsed, CPR gave any stranger the license to engage in prescribed actions to reverse the dying process. The rescuer should check the victim's breathing and, if no breathing can be detected, secure an open airway by tilting the victim's head back, and start mouth-to-mouth ventilation. Next, the rescuer should feel for a pulse, and, if lacking, begin chest compressions. From its establishment as the dominant resuscitation technique in the early 1970s, the efficiency of CPR has rarely been questioned and resources have been poured into constructing a community-wide "chain of survival"[1] that links every failing heart to the most advanced life-saving care possible in emergency departments.

While resuscitation techniques gained acceptance, an annoying problem remained unresolved: nobody could say how effective CPR was in saving human lives. The only data available were regional survival rates, but those varied widely—from less than one percent to 33 percent.[2] In most places, including big cities such as Chicago and New York, only one person in 100 would be saved on average while in Seattle about a third of resuscitative efforts would end up with a saved life. What explained such broad variation? Epidemiological researchers looking at the different survival rates could not compare them because no consensus existed about what counted as a true resuscitative effort (is every

1

attempt at reviving a resuscitation, or should only the cases with the best chance for survival be counted?), and how one should define survival (does survival mean that the patient walked out of the hospital, or does it include merely breathing?). The difference between one percent and 33 percent could be explained by varying methodological approaches, terminological and conceptual inconsistencies, the different emergency medical systems, demographic variations, the efficiency of CPR administration, or the quality of the resuscitative efforts. There was no conclusive way to tell why resuscitating in Seattle seemed vastly more successful than saving lives in Chicago.

In order to fix the confusing Tower of Babel that plagued emergency medicine,[3] international researchers gathered in the Utstein Abbey to propose a set of uniform guidelines to report outcome data for resuscitative interventions. Inspired by the International Committee of Medical Journal Editors, which recommended uniform requirements for articles submitted to biomedical journals, the researchers provided a glossary of terms, definitions for time points and intervals, a template for reporting data from resuscitation studies, definitions of outcomes, and recommendations for the description of emergency medical resuscitation systems. They published these standards aimed at "simplicity, conciseness, and practicality"[4] in the leading emergency medicine journals and requested the collaboration of journal editors and National Institute of Health peer reviewers to check for conformity to the Utstein guidelines. If every researcher gathers the data points suggested by the template and then uses the appropriate formula, policy analysts can now assess the efficacy of resuscitative efforts within and between emergency systems and better understand cardiac mortality. Recognizing that in the past "the cart was put in front of the horse,"[5] researchers will finally know after about thirty years of national education campaigns whether the point of diminished return is quickly reached in CPR, or whether more lives can be saved with, for example, automatic defibrillators.

The Utstein consensus conference is not an isolated instance of standardization in medicine. Over the past decades, a cottage industry of thousands of consensus conferences has emerged in the health care field, with psychiatrists attempting to standardize the assessment criteria for panic disorder,[6] transplant centers trying to reach consensus about national criteria for heart organ donation,[7] and manufacturers and users of ultrasound determining safety criteria of new devices.[8] In addition, national organizations, such as the American Heart Association, and international bodies, including the World Health Organization, regularly meet in umbrella conferences to update standard and safety guidelines related to the therapeutic use of biological products.[9] Standardization has penetrated every corner of contemporary medicine: it forms the foundation of collaborative international research protocols, medical information technologies, and reimbursement procedures.

Of particular interest in the current standardization movement is the emphasis on *evidence-based medicine* (EBM), or "the conscientious, explicit, and judicious use of current best evidence in making decisions about the care of individual patients."[10] Although evidence-based medicine means different things (including an orientation toward critical self-evaluation, the production of evidence through research and scientific review, and/or the ability to scrutinize presented evidence for its validity and clinical applicability), in common medical parlance it mainly denotes the use of *clinical practice guidelines* to disseminate proven diagnostic and therapeutic knowledge. The U.S. Institute of Medicine defines clinical guidelines as "systematically developed statements to assist practitioner and patient decisions about appropriate health care for specific clinical circumstances."[11] Such guidelines offer instructions on which diagnostic or screening tests to order, when to provide medical or surgical services, how long patients should stay in the hospital, and other details of clinical practice. Typically, a group of experts evaluates the scientific literature according to set criteria and then offers recommendations based on the strength of the evidence aimed at the practicing clinician.

According to the ideals of evidence-based medicine, clinical practice guidelines should be based on scientific evidence—preferably a meta-analysis of randomized clinical trials offering probability estimates of each outcome. Proponents of evidence-based medicine are wary of reasoning from basic principles or experience; they distrust claims based on expertise or pathophysiological models. They prefer to remain agnostic as to the reason why something should or should not work—rather, they objectively measure whether or not it works in real-life settings.

Yet such evidence is only rarely available to cover all the decision moments of a guideline. To fill in the blanks and to interpret conflicting statements that might exist in the literature, additional, less objective steps are necessary to create a guideline. A preferred method is the consensus meeting, in which experts, such as the Utstein resuscitation researchers, come together to discuss the contested issues and work toward a practically feasible recommendation. Such meetings have been criticized for the lack of transparency in decision making and the suspicion that the resulting guidelines are often as much the result of group dynamics during the meeting as of the scientific literature. Woolf et al. note that "the fact that a group of individuals think that a practice is beneficial does not ensure that it actually is."[12]

In response to such critiques, more systematic methodologies to develop practice guidelines emerged. Hierarchies to rate the scientific quality of the evidence upon which the guideline was based were developed, and statistical meta-analyses were used to aggregate critically the results of multiple clinical trials. In addition, cost-benefit data are increasingly being included in the evidence upon which the guideline is based. Relying on formal analytic methods and drawing from clinical epidemiology, guideline developers evaluate the benefits, harms, and costs of interventions and often derive explicit estimates of the probability of each outcome. Most guideline panels are comprised of health care professionals but occasionally also include methodologists, health economists, and patient and consumer representatives. Their task is to define a focus and an audience for the guideline; retrieve, evaluate, and synthesize the evidence; summarize the benefits and harms; and determine the appropriateness of the intervention.

For example, consider the guideline addressing the question whether screening for genital herpes should be part of a routine health care exam (see Figure I.1). Medical researchers estimate that 50 to 80 percent of American adults have type 1 herpes (HSV-1) while 21 percent have the second type (HSV-2). Yet the majority of people do not have a history of symptoms or outbreaks; the virus only shows up in blood tests.[13] Genital herpes is considered dangerous in people with weakened immune systems and for women giving birth. According to some obstetricians, an active outbreak during delivery might generate fatal complications and constitutes an indication for caesarean-section and preventive drug treatment (with acyclovir). Sometimes pregnant women with partners who have a history of herpes are counseled to use condoms or abstain from intercourse during pregnancy. The guideline addresses whether those preventive measures are indicated by the evidence of the scien-

Figure I.1. U.S. herpes screening guideline.

Screening for genital herpes simplex.

RELEASE DATE: 1996

MAJOR RECOMMENDATIONS:

The **strength of the recommendation** for or against a preventive intervention was graded as follows:

A: There is good evidence to support the recommendation that the condition be specifically considered in a periodic health examination.

B: There is fair evidence to support the recommendation that the condition be specifically considered in a periodic health examination.

C: There is insufficient evidence to recommend for or against the inclusion of the condition in a periodic health examination, but recommendations may be made on other grounds.

D: There is fair evidence to support the recommendation that the condition be excluded from consideration in a periodic health examination.

E: There is good evidence to support the recommendation that the condition be excluded from consideration in a periodic health examination.

CLINICAL INTERVENTION:

Routine screening for genital herpes simplex in asymptomatic persons, using culture, serology, or other tests, is not recommended **("D" recommendation)**.

Routine screening for genital herpes simplex infection in asymptomatic pregnant women, by surveillance cultures or serology, is also not recommended **("D" recommendation)**. Clinicians should take a complete sexual history on all adolescent and adult patients.

As part of the sexual history, clinicians should consider asking all pregnant women at the first prenatal visit whether they or their sex partner(s) have had genital herpetic lesions. There is insufficient evidence to recommend for or against routine counseling of women who have no history of genital herpes, but whose partners do have a positive history, to use condoms or abstain from intercourse during pregnancy **("C" recommendation)**; such counseling may be recommended, however, on other grounds, such as the lack of health risk and potential benefits of such behavior.

(Continued)

Figure I.1. *(Continued)*

There is also insufficient evidence to recommend for or against the examination of all pregnant women for signs of active genital HSV lesions during labor and the performance of cesarean delivery on those with lesions **("C" recommendation)**; recommendations to do so may be made on other grounds, such as the results of decision analyses and expert opinion. There is not yet sufficient evidence to recommend for or against routine use of systemic acyclovir in pregnant women with recurrent herpes to prevent reactivations near term **("C" recommendation)**.

DEVELOPER(S):

United States Preventive Services Task Force (USPSTF)—Federal Government Agency (U.S.)

Source: www.guideline.gov. Based on U.S. Preventive Services Task Force, *Guide to Clinical Preventive Services,* 2d ed. (Baltimore: Williams & Wilkins, 1996), 335–346. Used with permission.

tific literature. Its intended audience consists of health care practitioners wondering whether they need to screen for genital herpes.

The guideline first reiterates the criteria for evidence and then offers recommendations with varying degrees of certainty based on a review of the research literature by federal health researchers. The researchers found "fair" evidence to recommend against routine screening for herpes in asymptomatic people and pregnant women while there is insufficient evidence for any other more specific recommendations. Thus the available scientific literature was insufficient to suggest caesarean-section, counseling, or preventive drug treatment as standard interventions. But the makers of the guideline acknowledged that other factors, including consultation with experts in the field, might result in taking these preventive measures.

Evidence-based medicine has become a powerful movement that promises to change the content and structure of medicine and its allied professions. Indications of the impact of this movement are new institutions, such as the Cochrane Collaboration, the National Institute for Clinical Excellence (NICE) for England and Wales, and the U.S. Agency for Healthcare Research and Quality (AHRQ) (formerly the Agency for Health Care Policy and Research [AHCPR]); new journals, such as *Evidence-Based Medicine, Clinical Practice Guidelines Update, Best*

Evidence (a CD ROM), *POEMs (Patient-Oriented Evidence that Matters)*,[14] *Bandolier, Effectiveness Matters*, and *The ACP Journal Club*; recurring editorials in top medical journals such as the *British Medical Journal*, the *Journal of the American Medical Association, Annals of Internal Medicine*, and the *New England Journal of Medicine*; classical medical and nursing textbooks discussing the importance of evidence-based medicine; innovations in methodologies and criteria to gather and evaluate data; the surge of randomized clinical trials in medical research; and the rise of "causal pathways," "care plans," and "outcome research" to streamline and evaluate every aspect of health care. Even critics of evidence-based medicine have their own journal: *Journal of Evaluation in Clinical Practice*.[15]

Outside of the spotlight, other standardization processes continue, often interlocking with and being reinforced by the drive toward evidence-based medicine. For medical data to become comparable, for example, terminologies and communication routes need to be standardized, and technical standards have to be implemented so that the information systems of all these different parties can communicate smoothly.

Particularly in the past five years, the development of clinical practice guidelines has boomed: in the United Kingdom an estimated 2,000 guidelines are in varying stages of proposal and implementation.[16] In the United States, early estimates put the number of guidelines between 1,400 and 4,000, with currently about 1,000 new guidelines constructed annually.[17] The web-based U.S. National Guideline Clearinghouse (www.guideline.gov), produced by the Agency for Healthcare Research and Quality, in partnership with the American Medical Association and the American Association of Health Plans, currently contains 921 guideline summaries.[18] All throughout the Western world (and increasingly in third world countries as well), professional societies, public-sector agencies, research organizations, health care insurers, health maintenance organizations, and individual health care institutions are constructing and implementing guidelines.[19] In fact, the number of guidelines being produced by all these different bodies, in all these different countries, leads to a bewildering situation, in which there may be dozens of often overlapping and contradictory guidelines for any given condition or decision problem.[20]

To create some order, the U.S. National Guideline Clearinghouse includes only recently made or modified guidelines, authored by recognized medical bodies, government agencies, or plans. In the United Kingdom, NICE plays a similar role, creating new guidelines and improving relevant existing guidelines so that they "fulfill the NICE criteria for quality and content" (www.nice.org.uk). Besides physicians, nurses, insurers, physiotherapists, and dental assistants have all discovered the bandwagon of evidence-based medicine, nursing, physiotherapy, and so on. This raises the question of why there is such a great interest in standardizing medical care at this historical moment.

HISTORICAL ROOTS OF STANDARDIZATION

Evidence-based medicine is part of a wider movement to generate uniformity and quality control by streamlining processes. In the broader historical context, standardization forms a powerful vestige of modernism lingering in an increasingly postmodern world. The notion that predictability, accountability, and objectivity will follow uniformity belongs to the Enlightenment master narratives promising progress through increased rationality and control. "Modernity can be viewed as a process of emphasizing technological standardization and eliminating other established or culture-based standards. . . . Modern standard setting is characterized not by a change of *type* of standards, but rather by the specificity of the processes created to prescribe them, and by the multiplicity of standards, their ubiquity, and their formality."[21] Indeed, ever since Max Weber singled out the bureaucracy as the ideal typical organizational structure of the modern capitalist state, standards emerged as one of the hallmarks of rationalization. Through the abstract, written rules of standards, efficiency and control could be documented across diverse organizations. Standards specify how we work, how our technologies interact; they hold our sociotechnical societies together. Even military conflicts cannot be waged without basic standards: when American troops first landed in Kuwait, for example, before they did anything, they had to install the standard Volt.[22]

The rudimentary principles of the current standardization movement were articulated in the shifting economical field of the late nineteenth to the beginning twentieth century. Economic historians argue that the need for standards emerged when production processes and goods crossed geographical boundaries and business and scientific methods were counterposed to faith in community and tradition.[23] The classic example of the need for standardization is the integration of the railroad system. Two U.S. trade organizations, the American Railway Association and the Master Car Builders Association, adapted the standard gauge track in 1886 and standardized automatic couplers and air brakes in 1893.[24] Another impetus toward the standardization movement of the late nineteenth and early twentieth centuries was a preoccupation with safety. An early government-sponsored study of steam boiler explosions showed that many were due to a lack of standardization of the boilers and their parts.[25] While some of the early standardization efforts remained contested (e.g., the battle against the metric system at the beginning of the twentieth century), a consensus developed among engineers and entrepreneurs that not standardizing hurt business by generating waste, duplicating efforts, and creating bottlenecks in production. The standardization efforts took off when antitrust activists demanded that monopolistic firms increase their efficiency. In addition, the First World War legitimized standardization efforts when the government, with the support of President Herbert Hoover, issued mandatory specifications for war-related purchases. Hoover also organized the "Division of Simplified Practice," which developed procedures for cutting down on various sizes, varieties, and grades of commodities.[26] Efficiency through standardization became a national preoccupation in the prewar United States.[27]

While the industrial standardization movement of the early twentieth century took place, the U.S. medical profession reformed the medical schools and their curricula, and the *hospital standardization movement* tried to create a set of minimal requirements to which every hospital should adhere. The impetus for standardizing hospitals came from the realization that patients would no longer be cared for by their trusted primary physician but by a diverse team of consulting and referring medical specialists relying on the recently developed laboratory sciences and diagnostic technologies such as clinical pathology and radiology. Such an interdisciplinary approach implied that patients would need to be cared for in hospitals instead of at home, in turn requiring hospitals to relinquish the stigma of pauper, welfare institutions and reach out to middle-class patients. This standardization movement also fed off the fear that if physicians did not establish efficiency standards themselves, public officials might do it for them. An extra impetus was the desire and necessity to make hospitals financially responsible institutions.[28] The American College of Surgeons specified a number of standard hospital criteria needed for the proper care of patients, including specific case records, clinical laboratories, payment schedules, postmortem investigations, training procedures, and safety measures. Not every reformist proposal made it into the standardization movement. The parts of early reform proposals dropped included all efforts to evaluate doctors or limit the autonomy of individual hospitals. The parts that survived were well-organized medical records (see Chapter 1 for a detailed discussion), some form of staff organization, and access to X-ray facilities and a clinical laboratory. The American College of Surgeons began accrediting hospitals in 1919. "Control of the hospital was in the hands of medical men, and the method of control was standardization."[29]

A controversial outgrowth of the early standardization movement was Taylorism, or scientific management. Taylorism took a production process and improved the efficiency of the workers through time-motion analyses and a differential piece-rate system of payment. Evidence-based medicine is often (critically) compared to scientific management because of its focus on behavioral change with scientific underpinnings.[30] With a stopwatch in hand, engineer and former machinist Frederick W. Taylor would measure how long it took to perform the elementary movements of a job. For example, smoothing a wooden surface would be subdivided into smaller tasks: lift the piece from the floor to the planer table, level and set the piece, put on the stops and bolts, handle the mechanical planer, remove stops and bolts, remove piece to floor, and clean the machine.[31] Adding up the time units, including time for "unavoidable delays," generated a standard time in which to complete the job. This time could be improved if the manager eliminated the false, useless, and slow movements and used the standard time to calculate an incentive wage instead of paying workers a daily rate. For some kinds of work, the studies showed that regular rests and a shortened workday might increase productivity. Managers then taught the standard best method to employees and made sure that every worker could do the tasks of the person below and above him or her in the hierarchy.

Taylor's goal was to increase the productivity process while providing increased prosperity for management and workers, promising an increase in productivity and wages of 30 to 100 percent (the productivity increased more than the wages so that the average production cost went down).[32] But at the same time, he hoped to create a scientific base for managing employees by discovering the laws and principles of working. Taylor's vision of science was one of unsophisticated positivism mixed with engineering pragmatism: through rigorous observations engineer/scientists could discover laws of human behavior and then optimize them through modifications and incentives.

While one of Taylor's four principles of scientific management was to obtain "intimate friendly cooperation between the management and the workers,"[33] scientific management was largely perceived as a solution for labor problems. Taylorism subscribed to the notion that antagonistic management-worker relationships could be solved through crude early behaviorism. The problem was called "soldiering," or workers' ability to pace the work rate. According to David Noble, workers engaged in pacing to "keep time to themselves, to avoid exhaustion, to exercise authority over their job, to avoid killing so-called gravy piecerate jobs by overproducing and risking a rate cut, to stretch out available work for fear of layoffs, to exercise their creativity, and, last but not least, to express their solidarity and their hostility to management."[34] Scientific management was an attempt to transfer skills from machinists to the slide rules and instruction cards of management, changing rule-of-thumb management into its scientific counterpart.

This transfer did not materialize as expected by the corporate reformers. "No absolute science of metal cutting could be developed—there were simply too many stubborn variables to contend with."[35] Indeed, scientific management only caught on because large businesses, afraid that antitrust legislation would cripple them, considered novel means to become more cost-effective. When the railroad companies requested an increase in ticket rates, Louis Brandeis argued instead in a landmark legal case that the railroad's mismanagement had retarded their profits. Scientific management proponents testified that their methods could have saved the railroads $1 million per day. The court ruled in their favor. As a consequence of extensive publicity, "scientific management" became a household term[36] and under the efforts of Lillian Gilbreth it literally entered the household with scientific management cooking, house cleaning, and home economics. For example, she wrote:

> Like factory workers, children will be inclined to cooperate once they re-
> alize that their individual interests and skills have been taken into account
> in the management process. A household survey might reveal, for ex-
> ample, that one child is much more interested in washing dishes if she
> receives a new apron to wear while doing this task. Simple and low-cost
> adjustments such as this can be made to improve the cooperative spirit
> among family members and to make the home a happier place.[37]

After the momentum of scientific management slowed down with
changed labor relationships and management procedures in the after-
math of the First World War, standardization lost its broad ideological
appeal and disappeared from the public's attention. It became a mundane, practical matter of ensuring that fire hoses fit fire trucks, or that a
spare part for a car would match the original product's design. It was
nothing spectacular, and nothing that would arouse interest outside of
the backrooms where technicians elaborated their "minute specifications."[38] With the growth of international trade organizations after the
Second World War, however, standardization reemerged in the public
picture. Standardization appeared to be a highly useful means to avoid
direct political conflicts about barriers, inequities, and asymmetries in
international trade, and so a focus on standardization reemerged as the
"product of a global economy":

> If goods and services are to be freely exchanged across boundaries, given
> the complexities of multiple legal systems, the nature of the transaction
> [including what the purchaser can expect of the product] must be pre-
> cisely identified.[39]

Whereas scientific and technological progress provided the ideological
luster that was associated with standardization at the beginning of the
twentieth century, Krislov concludes, now standardization's appeal lies
in the ideology of the free, global market: standardization is viewed as a
necessity due to changes in the scale and complexity of commerce. Over
the past decades, the European Union has made standardization of basically everything tradable a top priority. Economist Peter Grindley puts
standards central to a successful business strategy, offering advice on
how to "win with standards."[40] He argues that in order to take advantage of standardization, businesses need to adopt counterintuitive economic practices, such as sharing proprietary technology, encouraging
standard adoption even if it generates more competition, and adopting
a technically unexciting design to increase the total size of the market.

The standard is here viewed as the base to accumulate complementary products and lock in customers. In order to gain a competitive advantage, consumer protection groups have seized the standardization process as a means to increase safety of products[41] while some government reformers have used their leverage in standard setting to force policies that would have little chance of succeeding via traditional legislative routes. California's air resources board, for example, has been a leader in setting fuel emission standards, requiring manufacturers to come up with cleaner cars.

In medicine, the overall interest in standardization similarly petered out after the first decades of the twentieth century. With the fading belief in the high hopes of scientific management, and with professional worries about the side effects of the standardization recipe (not the least of which was the never-ending threat of tight government control), it lost much of its original appearance. The licensing bodies continued their control of medical education and hospitals, but such developments were now no longer in the spotlight of the public's and the profession's attention.

In the late 1980s, standardization gradually reemerged as a focal point of interest in the health care field. In medicine, however, this did not initially take the connotation of globalization, strategic advantage, and free information exchange. Here other drives were at work. Whereas at the beginning of the twentieth century, standardization stopped short of prescribing the content of medical work, now this aim was at the heart of the increasing number of guidelines and guideline-creating agencies. Evidence-based medicine advocates wanted to intervene at the moment of a health care provider's special expertise: medical decision making. Earlier standardization attempts were almost always restricted to the skills, tools, and facilities required for that work: the required training, the required ancillary personnel, the design of the surgical theater, and so forth. The content of the work itself was left unaddressed: to decide the proper course of action for a given solution was the unique prerogative of the individual professional. Faced with a patient in situations that were never identical, the application of scientific knowledge was the art that only an experienced, true professional could master. Now, however, evidence-based medicine is foremost about delineating what sequence of activities constitutes a professional response to a given situation. Guidelines elaborate how scientific knowledge should be applied. Of all the kinds of standardization attempts that have affected medicine in the twentieth century, evidence-based guidelines represent the farthest-reaching and most direct attempt to prescribe and preset the actions of health care professionals. At the same time, evidence-based medicine also enlarges a conceptual space for other forms of standardization in medicine. Dovetailing on the success of evidence-based medicine, drug corporations have attempted to standardize drug delivery in novel ways, researchers have engaged in complex standardized international collaborative research, and government agencies implement welfare policies by streamlining standardized protocols to assess disability and workers' compensations.

The recent rise of guidelines has been championed by several major figures. In Britain, Archie Cochrane was captured by the Germans during World War II and became the medical officer to 20,000 prisoners of war. Because Cochrane had access only to the most basic medical tools to treat the starved and diseased patients, he expected many of his patients to die. To his surprise only a handful of prisoners died, mostly from gunshot wounds. During a later prisoner-of-war experience, Cochrane had more modern medical procedures at his disposal. Because mortality rates were much higher in the second camp, Cochrane feared that inappropriate interventions caused unnecessary deaths. In 1972, Cochrane published *Effectiveness and Efficiency*, arguing against medical overuse of techniques with questionable evidence. He made a plea for investigating medical interventions with randomized clinical trials. Services that were harmful, not effective, or overly expensive could then be replaced by underutilized better techniques.[42] Likewise, he argued for the urgency of systematic reviews of randomized controlled trials on a given topic, so that professionals would have quick access to high-quality summary information about the evidence for or against a certain intervention. The Cochrane Collaboration, named after him, now performs and collects such reviews, using state-of-the-art statistical techniques (www.cochrane.org).

In the United States, the work of epidemiologist John Wennberg made the need for more scientifically supported medical care blatantly apparent. For several decades Wennberg has been publishing the *Dartmouth Atlas of Health Care*.[43] This book maps the frequency of a variety of medical interventions by geographical area. The results confirmed an astonishing variability of medical practices depending on where the patient happened to reside. For example, the researchers found that a Medicare patient in early stages of prostate cancer was eight times as likely to have his prostate gland removed if he lived in Baton Rouge, Louisiana, than if he lived in Tuscaloosa, Alabama. In some parts of the country radical breast cancer surgery was performed thirty-three times as often as breast-saving lumpectomies. Higher surgical rates were almost perfectly correlated with the availability of surgeons and diagnostic tests; thus people who underwent angiograms (diagnostic tests for heart and artery blockages) were much more likely to undergo bypass surgery.

The great variation for almost any intervention could not be explained by chance but was born out of inadequate medical knowledge, physician practice styles, patient preferences, over-reliance on inadequately verified diagnostic tools, and basic inequities in the health care system. One of the proposed solutions to counter over-reliance on surgical fads was to provide a scientific evidence basis for hysterectomy, mastectomy, carotid endarterectomy, and other interventions in the form of clinical practice guidelines. Wennberg's retrospective studies of patterns of care helped establish optimal treatment levels. Particularly, government agencies (but also medical professional organizations) were interested in this research since it provided them with tools to check outcomes and allocate financial resources. Already in 1984, Wennberg urged a greater place for clinical epidemiology in academic medicine.[44]

A third figure associated with evidence-based medicine is David Sackett, who was born and educated in the United States but who built a career in Canada and the United Kingdom. As a clinical epidemiologist, Sackett developed research methods for testing medical innovations, for evaluating the scientific validity and clinical merit of medical interventions, and for educating physicians in applying the "current best evidence" from research. Together with Cochrane and Alvan Feinstein of the United States, Sackett made many methodological contributions to analyzing data gathered in the randomized clinical trial and legitimated clinical epidemiology as the foundation of evidence-based medicine. Sackett was instrumental in coining and promoting the term *evidence-based medicine* and articulating its principles.

These three major figures together with others have become identified as the founding fathers of the evidence-based movement, laying the groundwork for clinical practice guidelines as the solution for the lack of scientific working habits in the health care field. Yet why did the evidence-based medicine movement take off so strongly in the 1980s? Comparable ideas, guidelines, and tools had been around for a long time, but only in the late 1980s did they suddenly come center stage. Put briefly, the recourse to guidelines and the strain that this placed on the cherished individual autonomy of health care professionals has become necessary to legitimate the professional's claim to exclusive expertise in health care (see Chapter 3). Whereas 100 years ago the profession was at a position of newly established, unprecedented strength, after the second half of the twentieth century, its position had come under increased pressure. With spiraling health care costs, more emancipated patients/consumers, increasing attention to medical practice variations, an information overload, and an overall critical scrutiny of the role of experts and professionals in society, the medical profession felt it had to take unprecedented action to maintain its position as exclusive safe-keeper and wielder of medical knowledge. "Unexamined reliance on professional judgment," it is argued, will no longer do. "More struc-tured support and accountability for such judgment," in the form of evidence-based guidelines, is required to ensure the trust in the medical profession.[45] The crucial importance of taking the lead in these devel-opments is framed as a matter of professional survival: "What changes are implemented and how successful they are will depend on who takes the leadership role in developing guidelines: the profession, business, the government, or insurance companies."[46]

On the whole, these other parties all enthusiastically underwrite the importance of evidence-based medicine, creating a powerful network of allies and funding agencies propelling the movement. For govern-ments and insurers, evidence-based guidelines promise more insight into and openness about medical decision making, affording an in-creased grip on the primary care process and, concurrently, opening up a new means to achieve cost control. The same guidelines that explicate optimal decision-making procedures can of course be used to regulate those processes (to delineate reimbursable from nonreimbursable ac-tions, for example). For these parties, a promising option is to add eco-nomic evaluations to the evidence written into the guideline. Whereas evidence-based guidelines usually limit themselves to stating what di-agnostic and therapeutic actions are effective, with the help of health economics they can also provide evidence of the efficiency of these actions. Through cost-effectiveness analysis, for example, the costs of different interventions can be compared and weighed against their effects. In this way, by only underwriting interventions that are both effective and efficient, many policy makers hope guidelines can become a means to counter the never-ending increase in health care spending. Yet, it is not only cost containment that guides third parties. Nick Manning discusses how the U.K. government was instrumental in generating the research evidence and guidelines of a new personality disorder in order to allow preemptive incarceration.[47]

Patients and other health care professionals similarly tend to welcome the openness that comes with explicating decision procedures through guidelines. It allows them to be more informed partners in the interaction with physicians, and it brings the existing uncertainties in the medical knowledge base to the fore. In addition, other health care professionals see the creation of guidelines as a crucial strategy in their own professionalization process. By showing that they have a solid knowledge base, just like the medical profession, and that they are self-critical and scientific in their approach, these professionals hope to obtain high professional status.

Another development that weaves its course into the further growth of evidence-based medicine is the emergence of information technology in medicine. Dickersin and Manheimer note that "although science has long been acknowledged as the backbone of medicine, the actual practice of evidence-based healthcare may not have been possible before information systems technology advanced to its current state."[48] More specifically, the development of guidelines will merge with what has been labeled the "next major change" in medical record keeping after the introduction of the patient-centered record:[49] the replacement of the paper patient record by an electronic patient record. This development has taken off full force since the early 1990s, stimulated by national and international funding both in the United States and in Europe,[50] and driven by the same ideology that has driven international standardization after World War II: the notions of globalization and free information flow.

The diverse drives, developments, and parties involved make for a fascinating yet volatile mixture. The different aims are not easily reconciled: enhancing the patient's position might not be the most cost-effective option, and enhancing the payers' insight and control (through standardizing fixed courses of action, or through channeling information flows from the primary care process to the insurer's offices) may threaten the profession's position. These potential conflicts are real, and the further development and implementation of evidence-based guidelines will be the playing field on which these tensions will be played out. Although standardization in medicine has not become equated with the aims of globalization and free information exchange, as in the larger societal context, it has taken over the thoroughly de-politicized focus on technical measures that made standardization such a powerful phenomenon on the international political scene. In medicine as well, standards and guidelines can be discussed with regard to their scientific qualities or their technical adequacy, but to speak of their political nature seems almost to commit a category mistake.

RATIONALIZATION VERSUS REGULATION

> Evidence-based medicine is portrayed as an alternative to medicine based on authority, tradition, and the physician's personal experience. The role of politics is rarely mentioned. When discussed, politics is portrayed as what evidence-based medicine will avoid. . . . Changing medical practice requires the development of political, legal, and medical institutions that oversee medical care. Promoting medical practice based on evidence will therefore necessitate more, not less politics.[51]

The high hopes and pervasive skepticism surrounding standards indicate the contested nature of standardization. Some proponents of evidence-based medicine have gone as far as to label the recent standardization efforts in health care and evidence-based medicine a paradigm shift in health care[52] or even a new social movement.[53] Critics, on the other hand, have referred to evidence-based medicine proponents as "aerobatic children vaulting through the statistical stratosphere"[54]—emphasizing the theoretical void[55]—and have characterized evidence-based medicine as a "fundamentalist cult with evangelical tendencies."[56]

For supporters, the cost-benefit analysis of standardization is straightforward. Rigorous evidence-based medicine offers a tight link between medicine and scientific evidence, leading to better and more efficient care, improved health outcomes, better educated patients and clinicians, a scientific base for public policy, a higher quality of clinical decisions, and better coordinated research activities. It provides every interested party with accessible and simple information to evaluate the necessity, benefits, indications, harms, costs, and risks of a particular intervention. Because evidence-based medicine integrates clinical acumen with current best evidence, it makes the competent clinician even more competent and less likely to become blinded by experience or theorizing. Following Max Weber, advocates of standardization argue that the process is a sine qua non for effective communication and collaboration because it facilitates a transparent medical practice. Standards bring order to a modern world and facilitate coordination between diverse entities (medical specialties, hospitals, industries, and countries) without a centralized legal authority. Advocates argue that some level of standardization is necessary and inevitable for rational social action. The evidence-based medicine movement helps to move the health care field in the direction of an "exact science."[57]

Critics, on the other hand, charge that evidence-based health care turns clinical practice into bland and unsavory "cookbook" medicine. This overused metaphor suggests that health care providers would merely follow recipes, executing what others have decided, and would stop consulting their own intuition and experience. Behind a negative assessment of standardization lies the accusation that standards lead to watered-down competition, innovation, autonomy, and creativity, concocting a world of increasing and empty sameness. This "McDonaldization" of medicine resides in the standard approach to health care problems advocated by the guidelines, in which every patient problem would be addressed generically, as one more instance of the same.[58] In this way, it is argued, evidence-based medicine is bound to repeat the mistakes of scientific management. In medical education, clinical uncertainty might be managed by simple rule following, undermining the role of expertise and charismatic teachers. In medical practice, a clinician's prized autonomy might become secondary to what others have decided is best, resulting in the loss of individualized treatment. Standards, in this view, may become the unfair advantage that the powerful outsiders—managers, insurers, governments, and/or other professionals—impose on the powerless insiders. Worse, the traditional health care professions might be invaded and replaced by cheaper, less educated auxiliary occupations. Within medical subdisciplines, different professional groups formulating opposing guidelines or nomenclatures might create divisive internal strife and undermine the public's trust in health care. Critics also point to examples of "inefficient" standards, including a guideline for sleep apnea that because of its over-reliance on randomized controlled trials provided the wrong perspective on the disease, even missing the reason why it was treated.[59] Critics note that the goal of uniformity is undermined by the abundance of competing standards. Finally, critics have assailed the conceptualization of medical practice at the heart of evidence-based medicine, listed methodological problems in clinical trial research and in postulating from epidemiological data to clinical situations, and allege authoritarian motives under the guise of anti-authoritarianism.

The contested nature of standardization centers on its politics. The political heritage of standards is apparent in Taylor's promotion of scientific management as a behaviorist tool to solve labor problems, standardization as an alternative tool for governmental and legal antitrust actions, the deliberate positioning of private industry bodies, action groups, and government organizations to seize the standard-setting process, and the emergence of evidence-based medicine against the threat of third parties to regulate health care. Critics and supporters agree that standards emerge out of political concerns and can be used to implement or thwart regulation. But they disagree on the need for such regulation and the usefulness of standards as policy tools. The most often heard critique is that standards over-regulate. Standards undermine the expertise of professionals, constituting an unnecessary and harmful intrusion into a world of autonomous experts. Comparing evidence-based medicine to a "rationalistic dictatorship based upon simplistic and incomplete analysis," one critic states, "my cards are on the table. I see EBM, in its present form, as a dangerous delusion; erroneous in both rationale and conclusions, and a potentially lethal weapon in the hands of misguided regulators and reformers."[60] This critic reiterates a widespread fear that the payers in the health care system, governments and insurers, might regulate the health care field and hold it accountable using evidence-based parameters formulated by the professions.

Supporters point out that standards are necessary to safeguard professional autonomy and exclusive expertise because they constitute a form of self-regulation. While third parties might try to enforce standards through sanctions, a distinguishing characteristic of standards is that, in comparison to laws and directives, they remain impersonal and voluntary means of regulation. One of the great attractions and weaknesses of evidence-based medicine is that while experts might have decided what is best, it remains up to the professionals to acquaint themselves with the clinical guidelines and follow the consolidated advice. For supporters, the bigger threat to professional medicine is the great variability among care providers. They consider clinical practice guidelines an educational service to keep busy colleagues informed of the current state of medical knowledge. In their view, evidence-based medicine restores democracy to medicine. The basis of medical authority is not accumulated experience and credentials typical of seasoned clinicians but familiarity with scientifically validated knowledge. Clinical practice guidelines have the potential of leveling the medical playing field.

Dictatorship or great democratic equalizer? The pro and con positions with regard to standardization have been reiterated since the nineteenth century, leading to analytical gridlock. Two economists end their exhaustive review of the standardization literature with the disappointing admission, "we have no answer to the question of whether we need more or less standardization,"[61] and repeat that standardization requires more attention from social scientists, a claim echoed by others.[62] While it is indeed surprising how little attention standards have received, particularly in the field of medical sociology,[63] in this book we suggest a less antagonistic way of studying standardization. Instead of debating the advantages and disadvantages of standardization and getting stuck on a rhetorical level of analysis, we propose a study of the *politics of standardization in practice.*

Drawing from the interactionist sociology of work, science studies, and ethnomethodology, we are interested in how evidence-based medicine changes the practice of medicine on both a micro and a macro level. Opponents and supporters agree that standards provide order but disagree on the merits and need of such ordering. We ask instead: what is being ordered, who does the ordering, what is the difference, and how does it change medical care? Critics claim that evidence-based medicine stifles creativity and autonomy. We wonder what sort of autonomy health care practitioners had before guidelines were introduced to the hospital ward and what kind of autonomy they have after they structure their work according to guidelines. Advocates envision true democracy in health care, where the best science guides the hands of the practitioners providing similar care to a diverse patient population.

We question what constitutes the "best" science and explore under what conditions similarity, uniformity, objectivity, democracy, and universality are obtained. In this book, we bracket the claims about standardization and analyze what standards *do* in medical practice, investigating the changes obtained through standardization.

In our viewpoint, the politics of standards should not be located solely in the regulatory-political environment from which standards emerge but in the standards themselves. Standards are inherently political because their construction and application transform the practices in which they become embedded. They change positions of actors: altering relations of accountability, emphasizing or deemphasizing preexisting hierarchies, changing expectations of patients. It is in these transformations that we are interested. We thus propose a political gestalt switch: instead of focusing on whether the broader historical climate favors standardization, we will foreground standards as political tools.

Our approach rests on three tenets with methodological and theoretical implications:

1. *Situated knowledges.*[64] We follow standardization from the viewpoint of particular actors, recognizing that different agents would have experienced the same event differently. Every interaction is viewed as an intersection of multiple trajectories rendered meaningful from varying perspectives.[65]
2. *Blurred agency.*[66] Following a distinguishing characteristic of actor-network theory, we view standards as exerting agency in a particular situation with other agents: people and machines. While we assume that standards act in health care situations, the question remains what they achieve and how relevant their role is.[67]
3. *Emergent politics.* Standards are political entities because they reorder practices and change the position of different actors. They do not do so in and of themselves, but only as part of a network in which their own properties emerge with those of the human and nonhuman actors they affect.[68] One important aspect of these politics is power.[69] How power differences are transformed (or strengthened) through standards is one of our key points of interest.

These three tenets lead to a central empirical research theme: we focus on how the world of medicine is "remade and molded" through standardization.[70] We investigate how standards become part of the ongoing scaffolding of a medical infrastructure: opening up new construction sites where medicine will flourish and cordoning off other places. Our interest is in how standards create configurations of instruments and people, and in the process redefine what these groups, individuals, devices, and eventually, health care are about. In this view, *standardization is*, paradoxically, *a dynamic process of change*. The implementation of clinical practice guidelines or novel nomenclatures generates action and creates new forms of life. We do not, then, rally with the critics in bemoaning the loss of expertise that would occur through standardization. For us, the choice is not for or against standards. Standards are not one uniform thing, with one uniform effect. They help to bring into existence new ideas, entities, values, and even subjects for medicine (what Ian Hacking refers to as "kind making"[71]). Yet *different* standards do so *differently*. It matters whether psychiatric standards speak about homosexuality as a deviant category or not. Similarly, as Steve Epstein has shown, it matters how experimental and control groups for a clinical trial are constituted. Should they be as homogeneous as possible (which mostly means mainly white males) so as to have as close an equivalent of pure experimental material as possible? Or should they be explicitly heterogeneous (containing proportionate numbers of nonwhite subjects and females) so as to ensure that the findings of the trial generalize better over all these different subgroups in the population?[72]

Even the simple Utstein definition of the standard resuscitation survival rate takes a stance about which lives are savable. Based on the work of resuscitation pioneer Peter Safar, survival is measured as "the number [of patients] discharged alive [from the hospital] divided by the number of persons with witnessed cardiac arrest, in ventricular fibrillation, of cardiac etiology."[73] This seemingly innocuous definition has important implications. The facts that cardiac arrests need to be witnessed, patients need to have a particular heart rhythm, and the arrest needs to have a cardiac origin mean that the overwhelming majority of situations in which people perform CPR will not be included in the main survival rate. Some researchers have since estimated that 80 percent of resuscitative efforts are excluded.[74] Only the people with the best chance of survival are kept. Effectiveness of CPR as measured by the Utstein survival rate will thus be much higher than a survival rate where all attempts are used in the nominator. A high survival rate has implications for funding of regional and local emergency medical systems, the task packet and status of paramedics, the decision-making process of individuals considering advance directives, and ultimately the efficacy of CPR to save human lives.

Different standards, then, create different worlds—and it is these differences that we focus on. In this book, in other words, we locate the political opportunity for social change within standardization and not in the niches that seem to have escaped it.[75] This perspective requires us to investigate both the form and the content of standardization: to look at what is standardized, how it is standardized, what is included and what is excluded, what novel configurations of things and people are brought into being, and how much uniformity is actually achieved.

FOUR KINDS OF STANDARDS

The etymological root of the word *standard* implies power. Originally a standard referred to a conspicuous object (such as a banner) carried at the top of a pole and used as a rallying point, especially in battle, or as an emblem.[76] In themselves, standards are thus measures to which qualitative or quantitative values are assigned.[77] At this moment, not much is standard about standards. *Standards* and *standardization* are broad terms, differently defined, covering many entities, even when confined to the medical context. We define *standardization* as the process of rendering things uniform, and *standard* as both the means and outcome of standardization. In the most general sense, a standard refers to a measure established by authority, customs, or general consent to be used as a point of reference.

To create some uniformity in the many entities that fall under the standard heading, we distinguish four ideal typical categories of standards. First, standards may refer to what we will call *design standards*, which set structural specifications: defining, for example, the properties and features of X-ray devices, the constitution of hospital resuscitation teams, the size of hospital beds, the jurisdiction of care professionals, and the sizes of injection needles.[78] Such standards are explicit and more or less detailed specifications of individual components of social and/or technical systems, ensuring their uniformity and their mutual compatibility. Without such supported standards, the 27 gauge 3.5" needle might not fit a syringe, professionals would not know who to consult, X-ray images or resuscitation rates from different hospitals would not be comparable, and huge supplies of linen would have to be kept, fitting many different bed sizes.

A second category of standards concerns *terminological standards*, such as the International Classification of Diseases (currently in its 10th version), the English Read codes for coding patient conditions and medical events, North American Nursing Diagnostic Association (NANDA—a coding list specific for nursing diagnosis), and the Utstein definition of the standard resuscitation survival rate.[79] Such classification schemes may be more or less formally structured, and may differ in scope and granularity. They are to ensure stability of meaning over different sites and times, and are essential to the aggregation of individual health care data into larger wholes. Statistical overviews of causes of death, searches in library databases (such as Medline), and practices of managed care all would be impossible without the ubiquitous presence of such terminological standards.

The third category of standards is *performance standards*, setting outcome specifications. For example, a performance standard can prescribe a certain maximal level of complication rate for a specific operation or a minimal score on an examination. Performance standards are often used to regulate professional work, since they do not prescribe what has to be done, or how something should be done, but only what the result of the action should be. In addition, performance standards are often used in technological design as an alternative to design standards. Mutual compatibility between different components can also be accomplished by precisely presetting the activities occurring at the interface between the two components, and leaving the processes and structures that result in these activities unspecified.[80]

The fourth and final category of standards is *procedural standards*, specifying processes. These are the clinical practice guidelines (practice policies or protocols) that we mentioned above. Such standards delineate a number of steps to be taken when specified conditions are met: how general practitioners should proceed when they suspect a new case of diabetes, what steps a nurse should follow in preventing decubitus ulcers, and what checks the custodians should perform before declaring an operation theater ready for use. These standards may be written by a single individual or produced through an elaborate process of literature analysis, statistical meta-analysis, cost-effectiveness studies, and consensus-building. They may be more or less detailed, more or less wide in scope, and focused on individual practitioners or on different cooperating professionals. They may restrict themselves to indicating what should be done, or focus in detail on how each step should be performed.[81]

Although terminological, design, performance, and procedural standards necessarily intertwine, procedural standards are the main focus of our analysis because these standards boost the stakes of standardization to the highest level and form the heart of evidence-based medicine. Such standards attempt to achieve the seemingly impossible: prescribe the behavior of professionals. These standards bring people from different disciplines and backgrounds together with a variety of diagnostic and therapeutic techniques and instruments. They are simultaneously the most difficult to achieve and the most contested. As we will see in more detail later, practice standards raise issues about human autonomy, flexibility, creativity, collaboration, rationality, and objectivity. In short, they reflect important cultural assumptions about how people live and work together.

In medical lingo, two additional kinds of standards repeatedly come to the fore. The *standard of care* is primarily a legal concept that refers to the level of medical care that can reasonably be expected from a skilled practitioner in a particular situation. It is defined as a minimum standard to which health care providers need to adhere to avoid negligence, and it can encompass design, procedural, and performance specifications. Such standards evolve depending on what is acceptable in a medical subspecialty in a specific region. Some rural hospitals with limited equipment will be kept to a different standard of care than large university teaching hospitals. In emergency medicine, lawyer William Ginsburg argued that electric defibrillation should be the standard of care during sudden cardiac arrest occurring outside hospitals. He supported his position with literature reports, official positions of professional emergency organizations, expectations of the general public, and juries in courts of law.[82]

The *gold standard* represents the ultimate standard in medicine. The notion of a gold standard was imported from the financial world. Countries linked their currencies in the nineteenth and early twentieth centuries to their gold reserves in an effort to provide unrestricted convertibility of other money into gold and to freely import and export gold in international trade.[83] In medicine, the gold standard is regularly used to describe definitive and decisive standards. For example, when discussing the decline of autopsies in hospitals, an observer noted that "the properly performed autopsy remains the gold standard of clinical practice."[84] Or when describing chronic fatigue syndrome, Aronowitz wrote that this condition "had no 'gold standard' diagnostic test (one that definitively identifies a disease, as a biopsy confirms cancer)."[85] The gold standard is thus the measure against which everything else will be measured: it constitutes the rock bottom to which new candidates for standards are compared, and it defines the truth. Gold standards, therefore, do not seem to evolve. Once they are put in place, their authority is so overwhelming that it looks as if they will resist time.[86] Currently, evidence-based medicine and the randomized clinical trial have become the new gold standards in the health care field. What counts as good clinical practice (and, more and more, what is reimbursable) is tied to guidelines based upon scientific evidence derived from randomized clinical trials.

Layout of the Book

In the first chapter, we go back to the beginning of the previous century to look at the activities of the first major standardization campaign in Western medicine: the U.S. hospital standardization movement. More specifically, we look at the efforts undertaken to introduce proper, patient-centered record-keeping procedures in U.S. hospitals. We delineate continuities and discontinuities between these activities and the evidence-based movement that came up almost a century later, and we further elaborate the way we tackle the topic of standardization in this book. One central conclusion of this chapter is that standards are inevitably political in nature in at least two ways. First, their construction process can be typified as a political process of negotiations and struggle between different stakeholders. Second, standards restructure the environments of which they become a part: reshuffling responsibilities between and within professional groups, redefining the patient, resetting relations between health care managers and health care professionals, and so forth.

In the second chapter, we focus on procedural standards and discuss what it is that such standards do in health care work. What is their impact on the everyday activities of doctors and nurses? We return to the theme of the world making of standards, and discuss how standards can be seen to simultaneously afford as many new skills and capacities as they endanger. At the level of the work itself, it is crucial to not remain stuck in a discussion for or against standards, but to focus on the content of the standard and the way it has been designed and implemented.

In the third chapter, we zoom in on the topic of professional autonomy, and tackle the charged love-hate relationship between professionals and standards in general, and clinical practice guidelines in particular. We focus on the different ways in which evidence-based guidelines present themselves as double-edged swords for the professionals and professions that encounter or generate them. We discuss the complexly interwoven relations of guidelines, clinical and professional autonomy, the compliance of physicians with these guidelines, and how all these issues are themselves interwoven with the ongoing attempts to open up the health care professions to external, third-party accountability.

Chapter 4 continues with this theme, but focuses on a specific case to spell out the issues in somewhat more detail: the introduction of guidelines in insurance medicine in the Netherlands. We study the way insurance physicians defined and perceived these guidelines, and how it affected their clinical and professional autonomy. This chapter brings two additional features into the analysis that are also importantly at stake in the introduction and use of standards. First of all, we focus on the role the notion of objectivity, of the scientific character of medical work, played in these developments. Second, we focus on the way the patient was defined in these guidelines. Different standards, we argue, not only affect professionals and professions differently: they may embed different notions of objectivity or of scientific medical work, and they can constitute significantly different patients.

The fifth chapter investigates the role of evidence-based medicine in medical education. Advocates of evidence-based medicine claim that the new paradigm will level the playing field, meaning that clinical decision making should depend on what the evidence says instead of on the experience of the senior attending physician. In addition, clinical practice guidelines should eradicate most of the clinical uncertainty faced in medical training. Based on interviews with residents in evidence-based medicine programs, we show that the incorporation of evidence-based medicine did not remove clinical uncertainty and the reliance on experience in decision making but instead reshuffled knowledge hierarchies and introduced new kinds of uncertainties.

In the final chapter we discuss the standardized rehabilitation of a highly charged medication: thalidomide. Thalidomide was a "horror" drug that caused a wave of birth malformations in the 1960s. Currently, the same compound is considered a promising treatment for a long list of devastating conditions, including HIV wasting syndrome and many cancers. The chapter discusses how the American federal drug regulatory agency and the drug manufacturer in collaboration with several other groups normalized the risk of thalidomide. At the core of the normalization was a new restrictive standard for drug distribution. This chapter centers on the negotiation and creation of standards before they are implemented and on the redelegation of risk within this configuration.

Each chapter is based on a different research project that one of us undertook during the late 1990s. Our methodology consisted of either in-depth interviewing, participant observation, or document analysis and followed sociological qualitative research standards. This means that for interviews, we sought informed consent, asked open-ended questions, and taped and transcribed the interviews. In the cases of participant observation, we introduced our project at a team meeting, answered all questions regarding our presence and confidentiality, and took field notes that were later transcribed. All this empirical material, including the documentary data, was coded and written up in memos following the grounded theory tradition pioneered by Anselm Strauss and Barney Glaser.[87] Our analysis, however, was not purely inductive or geared at concept development but was aimed at a dynamic engagement with the social science literature on standardization from an STS (science, technology, and society) and medical sociology perspective. We discuss the details of our methodology in the notes of the corresponding chapters.

1 Standardization in Medicine in the Twentieth Century

The Emergence of the Paper-Based Patient Record

> Hospitals existing, then, for the patient, his cure, his relief and the only means to this end being the medical profession, the standardization of hospitals must mean simply this—seeing to it that the highest possible percentage of the best medical knowledge and skill available in a community reaches the patients in the hospitals of that community.[1]

Ordinary patients who had been admitted to one of the leading U.S. East Coast hospitals in 1900 with a broken leg might have spent some six weeks there, receive no X ray (although the equipment would often be available), and have their urine tested only at admission.[2] One or two entries might be found in the record of the ward to which the patients were admitted. At admission some medical history, the nature of the fracture, the result of the urine test, and the mode of treatment might have been written down in a few sentences, and several pages later a remark might be found about the current state of the healing leg.[3] Attending physicians would have checked them maybe a few times more during their six-week stay, but such visits were rare.

Well-to-do patients would have been treated in their own rooms, equipped with nice beds, wooden floors, better food, and a private nurse. They might have received even fewer tests, because they most certainly would not be bothered with unnecessary interventions that were for teaching or research purposes. Yet they would have seen their physician (and only this one) frequently.[4] In this case, one might not find any entries in the hospital's records at all: the only notes, if any, might be found in the physicians' own notebooks, which they would keep in their offices.

At the turn of the twentieth century, wards, laboratories, and physicians kept their own casebooks. In the Mayo Clinic, for example, each laboratory, each attending physician, and each (outpatient) surgeon kept their own leather-bound ledgers.[5] These ledgers were a kind of log, in which notes about patients and patient visits were written down in chronological order, and in the terminology the individual physician saw fit. In the Mayo Clinic's outpatient ledgers, four or five case histories were usually entered on each page. In 1900, one such case history reads as follows:

> Oct. 17 [name, address] . . . Early widow for 6 years. Menses reg somewhat increased for past 6 months. Felt well until 3 months ago. Noticed an enlargement on left side. Once after flowing a good deal it seemed smaller 2 months ago.
> Diag: a tumor the size of a child's head either from cyst or soft fibroid.[6]

It is difficult to imagine from our current point of view, but these casebooks hardly played a role in the clinical care process. Doctors might keep their own personal reminders in diaries or on slips of paper, but because they would often be the only physician seeing a private patient (and because not much would happen to a patient on a poor patients' ward), much could be done from memory. The casebooks were kept for administrative, teaching, and research purposes.[7] They were mostly not even kept on the ward or at the site of care, but on a specially designed stand in the physician's personal office.[8] The records would often also be filled in after the case had already been dealt with. The "progress of medical science" was a more important reason for keeping records than the everyday care on patient's wards[9]—and, we might add, this is also true of the X rays and urine tests that were performed on nonpaying patients. The clinical care for poor patients on the regular wards was attractive to physicians not because it generated income (only private patients did), but because the steady stream of cases offered prestigious teaching and research opportunities.[10]

Within a few decades this situation changed radically. The use of blood and urine tests proliferated, and visualizing technologies such as X rays and endoscopic techniques became routine.[11] Such technologies had become part of medical training, and for the new generations of doctors they embodied the newly emerged, truly scientific status of medicine. During this period the status of these tests shifted from a marginal addition to clinical work to the necessary condition of medical diagnosis.

With these new technologies, the hospital's organization had also become complex: it now included separate pathological, photographic,

X-ray, and dietary departments and services, and one or more separate laboratory facilities. In 1900, patients would seldom leave their rooms: in some hospitals surgical interventions sometimes still took place on the common wards. A few decades later, however, both private and poor patients would be wheeled through the hospital, from service to service. New medical specialties emerged—radiologists, laboratory clinicians, pathologists—and separate billing procedures and bureaucratic routines came into being to handle this increased mobility, and to turn the hospital into a "modern, professional institution."[12]

These technological and interdisciplinary changes coincided with a thorough transformation of the medical record. From a bound casebook in the physician's private office, with handwritten notes gradually and consecutively filling the empty pages with descriptions of the working day, the record became a patient-centered casefile. All patients now had their own standardized records, which usually consisted of a binder or folder. In this folder we would now find the doctor's and nurses' progress notes (still handwritten) and, in consecutive sections, correspondence with the patient or about the patient, and standardized forms and graphs from the different laboratories and other auxiliary services. The record would be empty at the beginning, and slowly fill up with loose sheets, each new sheet added to its own section in chronological order.

In this chapter, we focus on the introduction of the patient-centered record in U.S. medicine at the beginning of the twentieth century. The introduction of scientifically sound record-keeping procedures was one of the central targets of the Hospital Standardization Program initiated by the American College of Surgeons. The program attempted to ensure that the "highest possible percentage of the best medical knowledge and skill available in a community reaches the patients in the hospitals of that community."[13] The program's initiatives, merging with hospital administrators' concerns for efficiency, led to widespread changes in the shape and content of U.S. health care practices, which were not always equally appreciated by medical professional bodies elsewhere in the Western world. In the Netherlands, for example, the U.S. focus on improving record-keeping procedures was seen as commendable, while the perceived emphasis on the standardization of medical work was felt to be highly problematic.

Our aim in focusing on these turn-of-the-century developments is twofold. First, this story puts the current emphasis on standardization and evidence-based medicine in historical perspective. The notion that standardization of medical activities is a necessary condition for the rational and optimal delivery of medical care appears to be at least a century old. This does not mean that the aims and hopes that are attached to standardization attempts have not changed: we trace some of the shifting purposes and forms of standardization that we see in the hospital standardization developments, and later in the emergence of evidence-based guidelines. At the same time, some features continue to be the same throughout the various attempts to standardize medicine. One of these common features is the apparent resilience of the problems at stake. The opening quote of this chapter is almost a century old, yet the need for standardization to ensure the widespread delivery of optimal care sounds remarkably like a *cri de coeur* from the evidence-based medicine movement.

Second, we draw upon this history to refine our theoretical points of departure. The introduction of a novel form of record keeping seems to be a small and modest intervention in medical work, yet it encompasses all four types of standardization we mentioned in the introduction (terminological, procedural, design, and performance standards). It would seem to require only the simple substitution of casebooks for casefiles: it appears to be a minor change in administrative routines, perhaps at most forcing more time to be spent on this least interesting part of medical work. The history told here, however, illustrates that the innovation and standardization of record-keeping procedures implies the thorough transformation of both the practices involved and the standards introduced. Processes of standardization, it will become clear, do not themselves follow a standardized, uniform path. The large number of elements involved, and the concurrent presence of multiple actors attempting to pull the developments in different directions, ensure that the trajectory of the development is jagged and unpredictable. In addition, this brief history of the patient-centered record illustrates that standardization processes are not merely technical and neutral events. Different standards bring along different worlds. They reconfigure the health care practices involved, and thus directly touch upon political issues: they reorganize the system of health care professions (shifting the autonomy of physicians), have important financial consequences, alter the lives of patients, and affect the position of hospital administrators.

This chapter zooms in on closely interrelated changes in the medical profession, in medical institutions, in the proliferation of new investigative and rationalizing technologies, and in the organization of the medical record. It draws upon historical research about late-nineteenth- and twentieth-century medical practice, and upon contemporary medical and hospital administration literature. It focuses mainly on the medical record and the medical profession (thus paying little attention to nursing records, for example), because this area is much better documented. In addition, the first part of this chapter mainly focuses on U.S. developments. Although many of the early roots of the modern, scientific hospital can be traced back to eighteenth-century Parisian and nineteenth-century German medicine, the specific twentieth-century complexity of the hospital organization, and the explicit discussion and implementation of novel record-keeping methods, occurred first in the United States, and then spread to Europe.[14] Hospitals in Europe followed suit in remarkably similar ways.[15]

"A Splendid Gain in Efficiency": The Emergence of the Patient-Centered Record

Hospital standardization, properly understood in its motives by both parties to the project, administered in a spirit of toleration and common sense, and accepted in a disposition of willing cooperation, cannot but result in a splendid gain in the general efficiency of the hospitals of this country. The high position of the national bodies supporting the movement, the character and personality of the men having most to do with its inception and its conduct guarantee the honesty and fairness of its principles as well as the prudence of its administration.[16]

Many historians have described the beginning of the twentieth century as crucial in the history of American medicine. It was during this time that the hospital obtained its pivotal position within U.S. health care. From a shelter for poor, sick inmates, it was transformed into a prestigious institution, where high-quality medical care based on scientific principles and technological innovations was delivered by professional caregivers.[17] Whereas in a country such as the Netherlands the "home physician as trusted counselor" remained in a central position,[18] in the

United States this central position was taken up by the emerging modern hospital.

Likewise, it was during this period that the American Medical Association (AMA) managed to firmly establish its professional position. A key process in this consolidation of the medical profession was the standardization of medical education. In the mid-1800s, a burgeoning system of commercial medical schools churning out diplomas to anyone who could pay tuition created a vast supply of cheap doctors, undermining the professional aspirations of their higher educated fellow physicians and threatening their economical position. These developments, and the extremely critical analysis of medical schools in the Flexner report in 1910, led the AMA to set minimum standards for medical schools. The number of required courses grew, and the curriculum became founded in biology-based medical research. The AMA's reform of medical education resulted in the concentration and homogenization of the educational system, a decrease in the number of medical schools and the number of licensed practitioners, and an overall consolidation of the AMA's professional authority.[19]

Like the AMA, the American College of Surgeons (ACS) had also been attempting to enhance the homogeneity and status of their profession. As in the case of the AMA, they opted for a centralized approach. One of their strategies was to set national, uniform criteria that would distinguish the "Fellows of the College" from "the lazy and ill-trained surgeons of your community."[20] To investigate and compare the actual treatment results of surgeons, they had requested morbidity reports of surgical patients from all over the country. Neither surgeons nor hospitals, however, appeared to have records that could be used for such a purpose. Attempting to compare surgeons or institutions, the committee had to conclude, was useless:

> A comparison of the morbidity reports of many of the best institutions in this country has convinced us of the futility of the great labor and expense which has been expended on them. Owing to diversity of methods of classification they are not comparable except in the most gross way. Some are arranged by disease alphabetically, some by regions, and others by elaborate systems modeled after the International List of the Causes of Deaths.[21]

Hospitals with general record-keeping procedures were rare, and even in the best institutions, the required data would have to be found in casebooks that were scattered throughout the hospital. To trace a patient's illness trajectory in such a situation, one would have to find all the entries that were dispersed both within and between casebooks. Sometimes, indexes were kept, through which individual cases and instances of a particular disease could be found—but such indexes were themselves highly idiosyncratic and often only usable by the individuals who had made them. Physicians would often keep their notes on loose sheets, or write down a few keywords in a notebook—or not keep records at all:[22]

> The ultimate benefiting of the race, the lessening of disease and its more efficient alleviation through medical research are justly coming to be regarded as the most profitable type of benevolent investment. And the charitable hospital that neglects opportunities to advance medical science is like the manufacturer who throws away valuable byproducts. That the great majority of American hospitals are following such a short sighted policy of neglect is truer, I believe, than is generally appreciated. . . . For want of sufficiently accurate, complete and accessible data, a vast amount of useful material is constantly thrown beyond the reach of those in the future who would utilize it.[23]

In addition, the circumstances under which surgeons worked were so variable that a comparison between morbidity reports would be meaningless. Some hospitals would possess new, aseptic, and electrically lighted operation theaters, while other hospitals had an operation room that would look much like an ordinary ward—including the fleas, the crowds, and the dirty floors and beds. Some hospitals had trained personnel to assist during surgical interventions and autopsies; other hospitals lacked such personnel.[24]

The college decided that they could only guarantee high-quality surgical care by setting minimal standards for the hospitals in which their surgeons worked. A contemporary observer summarizes the college's criteria as follows:

> A patient entering a hospital approved by the American College of Surgeons believes that he is protected against fee splitting doctors;[25] that in this hospital there will be X-ray and laboratory facilities, and all the scientific equipment and apparatus necessary to treat the disease with which he is afflicted; that a clean, well lighted operating room with expert graduate nurses in charge will be available if an operation is needed; that a complete record will be kept of all the findings and that they will be available if necessary for future reference.[26]

One of their core criteria was the presence of complete, accessible, and accurate records for all patients, which had to be kept by the hospital rather than by the individual physician:

> Accurate, accessible, and complete written records must be kept for all patients and should include patient identification, complaints, personal and family history, history of present illness, physical examination, record of special examination such as consultations, clinical laboratory and X-ray results, provisional or working diagnosis, proposed medical or surgical therapy, gross and microscopic findings, progress notes, final diagnosis, condition on discharge, follow up and in case of death autopsy findings.[27]

This change in record keeping is often heralded as an important move in the emergence of a medicine based on science: it thoroughly facilitated scientific research, and it symbolized the fact that medicine was organized around the patient rather than the individual doctor or ward.[28] Especially the former benefit was stressed in the many articles that now suddenly addressed "the record" in the medical literature. The importance of well-registered clinical information is crucial for clinical research, authors argued:

> In a way it marks the beginning of real clinical science, for each operation or each attempt at any other form of curative treatment in any hospital is an experiment. It seems curious that these experiments should not be recorded in most hospitals. Often the facts thus obtained would be of the greatest scientific value.[29]

In comparison with case histories distributed through casebooks, the patient-centered file offers a much easier and more efficient access to individual patient histories.

Such records, moreover, would allow professional self-control. "Ill-trained" surgeons could be weeded out from the worthy ones:[30]

> The advantage of having a complete hospital record such as Dr. Bottomley speaks of, not a long one, but a complete one, was illustrated to me. . . . [The superintendent of a large municipal hospital had received a complaint that the performance of one of his physicians, Dr. So-and-So, was not satisfactory.] The physician in question was told of the affair . . . and became very angry and said that he was being persecuted; that his results were just as good as anybody else's. Meanwhile the superintendent . . . had asked [his] clerk to take the records of four men occupying similar positions on the staff, the man in dispute being one of them, and bring him these men's records of operations for three months, the character of the operation, the result, and the number of days the patient remained in

the hospital, so that when this man came to him and said he was being persecuted he had definite facts to show that his death rate was high, and that the average length of stay of his patients in the hospital was longer than any other man's.[31]

For the college, however, these standardization attempts served more ends than the enhancement of the scientific nature of surgical work and the possibility to judge individual surgeons. Importantly, by focusing their standardization attempts on the operation of hospitals rather than the activities of surgeons, they attempted to increase their influence on hospital management. Slowly but gradually, medical professionals took over the management of hospitals from lay community leaders, and thus increased their control over the flow of patients through the hospital. By focusing on the doctor's setting and education rather than on the doctor's own performance, the ACS strengthened this development: they set criteria for quality that effectively enhanced their sphere of influence in hospitals without impinging on the individual doctor's clinical autonomy.[32]

Yet the college's focus on adequate record keeping did not in itself pave the way toward a patient-centered record system. In fact, their first criteria spoke about proper record keeping in general—they did not delineate the patient-centered casefile as the preferred way of record keeping. As long as records were complete and contained a certain set of standard data, they fulfilled the ACS criteria. The step toward the patient-centered casefile was entangled with the spread of the principles of scientific management within hospitals, which was becoming very popular in industry during this period. This approach was brought into medicine not so much through the medical profession as through hospital administrators, who aimed to control costs and enhance operational control over their increasingly expanding organizations. As a core part of the principles of scientific management, modern record keeping was both a response to and a prerequisite for the increase in the number of patients treated, generating both patient information and organizational complexity.[33] The move from a bound casebook oriented toward research, administration, and teaching to a casefile primarily oriented toward patient care reflected a need to coordinate a growing number of people and events.[34] The case records defined and distinguished the organizational subsections of the hospital, and allowed their mutual collaboration: all information concerning individual patient trajectories was automatically "filed as they were created," in their proper section, in the single binder that stood for a single patient.[35] The patient-centered record was to medical work what the introduction of cost accounting was to hospital administration.[36] It afforded the overview and management of increasingly complexly structured units ("the hospital" and "the patient"), and it was the science that both physicians and administrators so craved.

An author of a study on record-keeping procedures in hospitals praised the benefits of such a system:

> The value and need of an adequate system of case records for every modern hospital is so well recognized and generally appreciated that it hardly seems necessary for me to dwell upon it here. . . . [T]heir paramount value is found in their direct service to the community. This community service is brought about in two ways. First, through the study of methods and results as shown in the records, the hospital is able to give better and more efficient service, and, second, by giving convincing evidence of efficiency and an available measure of its service the hospital can seek and obtain more confidence, respect, and generous financial support and thus extend its scope and increase its ability to serve.[37]

The existence of adequate case records, this author argues using the favorite terminology of scientific management, is a "measure" of the hospital's service, and gives "evidence" of its "efficiency." An early textbook of medical record keeping nicely sums this up:

> The basis of this standardized service is to know what the hospital is doing, and to record its work in such a way as to enable an appraisement to be made of it. . . . Records, therefore, are a prime essential in any program of hospital standardization. . . . Case records are the visible evidence of what the hospital is accomplishing. . . . Not to maintain case records properly is like running a factory without a record of the product.[38]

Throughout offices in the United States, loose, subject-centered files were replacing the bound books in which administrators had been writing their reports. Files of documents "arranged by subject or by name became the generally preferred way to permit administrative documents to accumulate."[39] Just like letter books with chronologically stored in- and outgoing mail were replaced by vertically stored, loose files arranged by subject, and just like employees and nursing pupils each acquired their own records, the casebook was replaced by the patient record.[40]

The specific form that the patient-centered record took, then, has to be seen as the contingent merging of professional reform initiatives and the extension of principles of scientific management into the organization of hospitals. Through this interplay of drives (which were partly in conflict with each other—see further), the patient replaced the ward or the individual physician as the "unit" of the record. Rather than stemming from a contemporary humanistic desire to "put the patient centrally," it received an initial impetus as an attempt to enhance professional control over hospitals and over individual doctors. As much as signifying the progress of science, it was simultaneously a device crucial in the management of an increasingly complex organization and propelled by the urge to improve efficiency through enhancing management control. It made coordination between more and more actors feasible, and afforded overview and insight for physicians, hospital administrators, and community leaders.

Of Money, Bricks, and Marble: Achieving Standardization

> By certifying the surgeon as competent, certifying the surgery was unnecessary.[41]

The reformers, including both elite medical professionals and hospital administrators, attributed many benefits to the installment of proper and standardized record-keeping procedures in all U.S. hospitals. The actual achievement of this change in record-keeping procedures, however, was not an easy task. Hospital administrators, private patients, and physicians had to be persuaded, and a wholly new infrastructure had to be put in place for the creation and filing of these records. In a phrasing derived from current approaches in the sociology of science and technology, a network had to be created, linking doctors, administrators, records, and buildings in novel ways.[42]

Not all of these elements were easily enlisted. Practicing physicians, for example, at first did not have much to gain in changing their record-keeping routines. They had their own practices and patients, and patients would remain in the care of these private practitioners throughout their stay in the hospital. Such patients would not see many other doctors, and their patient data would be securely kept by their trusted, private physician. A personalized doctor-patient relationship was highly valued—and not just because this would ensure that paying patients would return to one's practice.[43] In such a situation, all a doctor would need were a few keywords in a personal notebook: the doctor knew his private patients intimately, followed them throughout the whole disease trajectory, and did not have to communicate with other doctors.

The poorer patients who populated the hospital wards were not fortunate enough to have a private physician who knew them through and through. Except from some initial tests, however, not much would happen to such patients during their stay in a hospital—and certainly not enough to warrant more than a few brief notes in a common ward record. For these patients as well, then, the existing record-keeping procedures were—ironically—adequate to the levels of care these "moral minors" could expect to receive.[44]

The reluctance of physicians to change their record-keeping routines, and to spend more time registering more information, was extensively criticized by the reformers. Medical record keeping, they argued, is characterized by "inexcusable laxity":[45]

> The various diagnostic procedures are often neither dated nor signed. . . . The bedside notes seldom give a complete picture of the case. There is likewise hardly ever a note as to the condition of the patient at discharge. . . . On one of the records there was found the following laconic account by an intern: "operation performed with alacrity, dexterity and celebrity."[46]

> Many a research worker in hospitals has had his ambition dashed to the ground, because upon undertaking a task that bore promise of extending even slightly our knowledge, he was confronted with incomplete, unsatisfactory and unreliable clinical histories—unreliable because entries concerning essential facts were poorly recorded.[47]

In addition to the increased efforts demanded from the physician, the calls for a patient-centered record were also contested by contemporaries because it equated private and nonprivate patients. Until then, records of private patients had been kept and owned by their private physicians. This ownership symbolized the unique relationship between doctor and patient, and the importance of trust and confidentiality: private information was something that should remain between the doctor and his patient. The ACS claim that record keeping should be the hospital's responsibility signified a breach in confidentiality that many physicians found unacceptable for their private patients.

Dr. Mayo, whose clinic first put into practice the patient-centered case file, commented ironically on such objections that he saw as resistance to centralized record keeping: "We hear objection sometimes to complete records for private patients . . . the poor have had records because, let us say, they could not help it; the rich and the middle class are just as deserving as the poor and they haven't the records."[48] In 1922 a public health committee lamented that private records were still often simply absent in the hospital's central record room: "The private patient records are worse than the ward records. In some of the hospitals, no records of the private patients are required for the central file, thus making the relationship of the patient to the hospital purely that of a hotel."[49]

This noncompliance of physicians was problematic because it could make it impossible for a hospital to fulfill the American College of Surgeons' criteria. In the study of record-keeping procedures quoted earlier, problems were indeed attributed to the stubbornness of the physicians:

> In response to the question of what difficulties were met with, not one hospital mentioned any trouble in getting the clerical part of the work done. The difficulties all seemed to be in getting proper reports of the histories, physical examination, operations, etc. . . . All this, of course, with the exception of the shortage of house officers, points to a lack of interest and cooperation on the part of the doctors.[50]

To ensure adequate record keeping under such circumstances, nurses were often asked to jump in: they could, for example, "help the doctor with examination, take his dictation, and record his findings."[51] As a more fundamental solution, hospitals started to hire new personnel to support the faltering doctors:

> Of course the first thing that suggests itself is to have a competent stenographer who will take down dictations at the time of the visit and after the operations. This stenographer could also take care of the clerical part of the work and the details of the follow-up system.[52]

In addition to stenographers, record clerks and record librarians were hired. The emergence of these new professionals signaled that the medical profession's emphasis on proper record keeping was slipping from their hands: the improvement of medical records systems was taking on a different shape than they had intended. The medical record librarians now established themselves as the guardkeepers of proper record keeping, ensuring a system that was optimally configured to the needs of a modern hospital—whether or not this corresponded to physicians' needs. Doctors complained about the proliferation of preformatted forms, in which they only had to fill in a few words or even just select a term from a pregiven list (see Figure 1.1). Such forms, they noted, shifted responsibility for the content of clinical work from the individual doctor to the system that developed and accorded the forms.[53] And indeed, statisticians and record officials started to scold physicians publicly for their poor record-keeping practices. They ridiculed doctors' fears of standardization:

> One realizes perfectly that any suggestion in the direction of standardizing case history writing, by the process of putting into operation methods which have been found sound and useful in other branches of science and in modern business, will at once be scornfully or even derisively received by some. It will be argued that any such process tends to cramp their individuality. This argument is perfectly valid. It will inordinately cramp such portions of their individuality as finds its expression in carelessness, inaccuracy, forgetfulness, and inattentive observation.[54]

Medical record officials defined themselves as the "watchdog of the hospital records"[55] and sometimes started to supervise doctors' work directly: "The record room clerk shall post each day on a bulletin board at the entrance of the hospital the number of incompetent histories opposite the name of the member of the staff responsible for their completion."[56]

The new professionals also became responsible for updating and enforcing adequate standardized medical nomenclatures.[57] The potential benefits of standardized, patient-centered record-keeping procedures could be reached only if medical terminologies would be standardized as well. If different physicians would use different terms for similar afflictions and interventions, results from treatments could never be compared, and communication between physicians would remain limited.[58] Some authors proposed fixed lists of permissible abbreviations, ward reference books, and nomenclatures outlining clinical procedures.[59] Several hospitals developed in-house classifications that suited their purposes best:

> The cards in the diagnosis catalogue are arranged according to Dr. Post's "Nomenclature of Diseases and Conditions," in which entries are grouped primarily under the different systems and secondarily under anatomical parts, in alphabetical order. Thus the cards referring to all the diseases of an anatomical part can be found at a glance.[60]

These new professionals were pivotal in ensuring the efficient functioning of the modern hospital according to the scientific management

Figure 1.1. Preformatted Physical Examination Form.

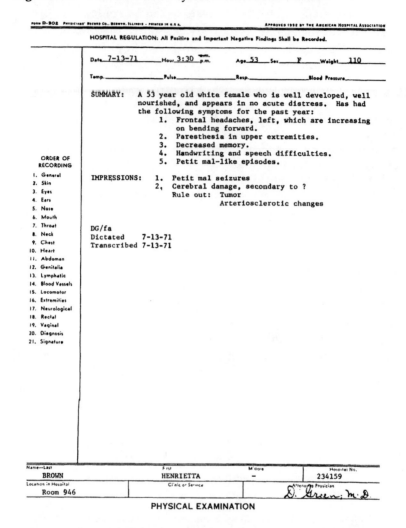

Source: Huffman, Edna K., and Elizabeth Price, *Medical Record Management*, 6th ed. (Berwyn, Ill.: Physicians Record Co., 1972). Reprinted by permission of the publisher.

ideals. Her (this was distinctly a woman's profession from the start) meticulous work, requiring precision and communication skills, would guarantee the upward flow of inscriptions:

> It is the record librarian who, reaching out to all parts of the hospital— to the X-ray department, the laboratory, the operating room and even to the home of the patient through follow up letters and with the aid of the social service department—gathers all the facts about every patient and makes it possible for the hospital superintendent to discover what kind of work his institution is doing. He gets his knowledge through the gathered statistics that make up the daily, weekly, monthly and annual reports of the record department. . . . If the record librarian is competent she keeps her finger on the pulse of the hospital staff.[61]

An unexpected side effect of the efforts to improve record keeping was that this made it possible for the records to acquire a legal function. Albeit not planned as such by the original reformers, this new function had a major impact on later developments. The legal function of health care records is all too obvious in our times, but at the beginning of the twentieth century their status was unclear:

> So called "bed-side notes" were not admissible in evidence. They were introduced during the examination of a hospital nurse, who was in the hospital at the time the plaintiff was a patient there. She describes the paper as a "temperature chart, known in the hospital as bedside notes," and said such notes were taken in each case where a patient was brought to the hospital. The court is not aware of any rule of evidence which makes such a paper, offered under such circumstances, admissible.[62]

Record keeping was too idiosyncratic and not institutionalized enough to serve as evidence: the Supreme Court ruled as late as 1933 that the charts and records brought to the Court in a particular case "were hearsay, self-serving and inadmissible."[63] Only when standardized record-keeping practices had become commonplace did patient records became fully accepted in court cases. The deindividualization of record-keeping practices—the institutionalization of procedures that made the records independent from the individual nurse or doctor who happened to record—turned the record into an objective representation of events. This record became the true record of a patient's condition or of a physician's actions:[64] "Subpoena of the record enables any court to obtain a true statement concerning the patient's care and treatment in connection with insurance claims, employees' liability claims, suit for damages and malpractice."[65]

The legal function subsequently became an important reason for further standardization of record-keeping procedures. As early as 1919, the importance of the record "in cases of tort, as a means for protection in suits for alleged malpractice, and in all other medico-legal controversies" was stressed as an important reason for adequate case records.[66] More and more, record-keeping procedures gradually became shot through with the awareness that every inscription in the record might end up on the desk of a lawyer or a judge. The importance of accountability has led to strict procedures regarding signatures and the completeness of forms, for example, and to rules regarding storage.

New terminologies, new personnel, a growing emphasis on accountability, and altered working patterns of physicians were not the only changes that the new forms of record keeping brought along. Hospital visitors toured the country, scoring hospitals' compliance with the ACS standardized criteria on standardized cards (see Figure 1.2). Hospitals were equipped with mechanical dictating and transcribing machines, under central supervision if possible.[67] Moreover, storing patient records on the wards or in physicians' offices was no longer feasible. Proper record-keeping practices now required the records to be stored in a central location within the hospital: the record room. To make a fast transmission of records possible, new technologies such as pneumatic tube systems could be installed.[68] However, more radical architectural changes were often necessary:

> In older institutions, . . . built before the days of hospital standardization or of emphasis upon hospital record-keeping, the installation of a record department has in many cases been a difficult problem. . . . The ideal record room is near enough to the operating room, laboratories, and staff room to make it convenient to access, yet sufficiently secluded to be a suitable place for quiet work, on the part of both the record room staff and the attending doctors, interns, and technicians who may come there to complete unfinished charts, for information, or for research.[69]

The emerging shape of modern hospitals, as centralized, multilevel structures, was partly due to the recognition that such architectural forms reduced the transportation times of the increasing circulation of paper, materials, and patients between wards: "Vertical transport is shorter than horizontal transport—although one remains dependent on the proper functioning of elevators and their operating personnel."[70]

The standardization of this novel record-keeping system, necessitating new personnel and investments in buildings and technology, was a costly and time-consuming matter. Although the hospital standardization movement emphasized that it did not intend "putting a premium on money, bricks and marble,"[71] many small hospitals (including many of the black hospitals) were not able to comply and disappeared.[72]

For European commentators, cost and time were not the only worrisome aspects of these U.S. developments. The Dutch medical profession, for example, was ambivalent. Commentators agreed with the need for complete documentation, and they were envious of the facilities created for U.S. physicians:

> While in our country, as far as I am aware, the doctor is expected to bring his own fountain pen and have a considerable passion for writing, the American doctor has more pleasant means at his service. Every hospital that carries any weight has a Record Department: a separate department for the treatment of disease histories. Young ladies, who not only have typing skills but who also know short-hand, are busy in there all day. They support all facets of administration.[73]

In the Netherlands, however, the architectural prerequisites for a centralized record-keeping system were highly problematic. Many hospitals were still built in European fashion: isolated pavilions, with a separate building for administrative functions.[74] Building modern, rational, and efficient highrise buildings, moreover, could run against many building regulations:

> In such [modern] hospitals, the gardens are endangered; not much remains of the demand we often encounter that every bed should be accompanied with 100 m² of grounds. . . . The Americans in general seem to have little regard for blooming flower beds and shrubs.[75]

More important, however, the Dutch physicians opposed the consequences of the American system for the position of the medical profession. In the Netherlands, it would be unthinkable to make the hospital the "guardian of the integrated patient data." The hospital was merely a "link in the chain of public health care," and this institution could never take the responsibility for the content and handling of patient information from the individual physician.[76] When Dutch authors spoke about standardization, they would refer only to matters of

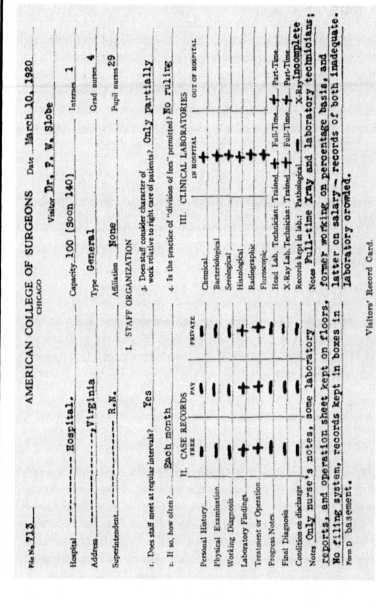

Figure 1.2. ACS "visitor's record card," on which the hospital visitor could score the hospital's compliance with the ACS standardized criteria.

Source: Reprinted from *Modern Hospital* 15:40, with permission from *Modern Healthcare*, Copyright Crain Communications Inc., 360 N. Michigan Ave., Chicago, IL 60601.

housekeeping (bedding, furniture) and financial administration (book-keeping methods and pricing). Clinical matters were to be kept out of this discussion.[77] The Dutch medical profession should guard against coercion and superficial schematism, it was argued, and it should be weary of the control on the "visits and work of the medical staff" that so typified the American system.[78]

When the Dutch Medical Association performed a study of hospital records much like the American College of Surgeons had done, their findings were similar but the conclusions were vastly different. This Dutch study became a news item in the *Journal of the American Medical Association:*

> The committee relates that in an examination of the books of the sixty-four hospitals in the Netherlands chaotic differences were found between the data recorded and the methods of compiling them in the different hospitals. Their records therefore cannot be compared, and thus are not a source for dependable statistics. The committee deplores this, and makes some suggestions which would remedy this state of affairs. In the first place, however, it deprecates any attempt to force uniformity in hospital records. The liberty of each institution to record and publish what seems to be important must not be interfered with. But certain data should be recorded, and these the committee thinks should be called to the attention of every hospital with the request to conform to the suggestions. The committee adds that the suggestions have been restricted to what is absolutely necessary, so as not to add to the *beslommeringen* of the hospital direction. (This useful and untranslatable Dutch word *beslommeringen* means "to involve in all sorts of difficult affairs.").[79]

In the face of similar variety in record-keeping procedures, the Dutch Medical Association stopped far from anything similar to a hospital standardization movement. The freedom of hospitals and physicians was not to be touched, and only a request to comply to minimal standards was issued.

STANDARDIZATION: FORMS, AIMS, AND CONSEQUENCES

> The man of business requires these standards for the sake of justice, the man of science requires them for the sake of truth, and it is the business of the state to see that our . . . measures are maintained uniform.[80]

The introduction of a new record-keeping procedure demands a thorough transformation of the health care practice in which this system is to function. The introduction of a seemingly simple administrative procedure involved the standardization of terminologies and the standardization of work processes of doctors and (newly hired) clerical personnel. Records had to be filled in standardized ways; communication patterns had to be standardized; and files were checked, stored, indexed, maintained, and retrieved in standardized ways. Authors advocated lists of permissible abbreviations to increase understandability of medical records, and some pleaded that clinical procedures had to be standardized as well (through, e.g., a ward reference book), so that doctors would know what exactly was meant and which technique was followed (e.g., when a functional liver test was ordered).[81] It equally involved many design standards, such as a uniform layout and size of forms, standardized storing systems for folders (Figure 1.3), a functioning pneumatic tube system, even a typical hospital architecture. Standardization processes depend on and trigger other standardization processes: as concentric circles of waves moving outward from the place where a stone has hit the water's surface, the standardization of record-keeping procedures triggered the emergence of standard file folders, which in turn triggered the emergence of standard folder racks and folder storing procedures.[82] Simultaneously, design standards were set for hospitals, performance standards were set for professional training, procedural standards were formulated for professional conduct (no fee-splitting, for example), and standardized accounting procedures were introduced and further refined.

What drove these different standardization efforts? Around the beginning of the twentieth century, the economist historian Krislov points out, standardization appeared to bring some godsend benefit for everybody. To standardize something—whether it was a nomenclature, a product, or a procedure, or the setting of a minimal expected performance—made it more effective and more efficient. It linked the object of these efforts and those undertaking the efforts strongly to the realms of science and technology, in whose progress managers and health care professionals, patients and community leaders all strongly believed.[83]

Beneath this underwriting of standardization as a common good, however, different parties had different views of just what constituted this common good. As we saw, the initiation of the hospital standardization program cannot be uncoupled from the ACS desire to enhance the

Figure 1.3.   Patients' histories, kept on the nurse's desk. "The desk is equipped with holding racks designed in such a way that each patient's name, inserted in a card on the holder, is clearly visible." (Cook 1927, 71)

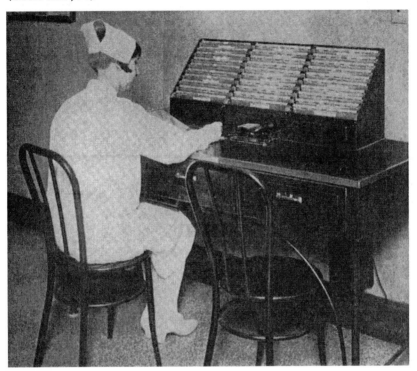

Source: Reprinted from *Modern Hospital* 24:69–72, with permission from Modern Health-care, Copyright Crain Communications Inc., 360 N. Michigan Ave., Chicago, IL 60601.

profession's position. The standardization activities helped eradicate "unworthy" surgeons, enhance the surgeon's working settings, stimulate self-improvement through improved record keeping and follow-up, and increased physician control over hospitals. Even those who were weary of the potential side effects of such a program admitted that the profession's lead in these matters was crucial: "it is wise that we lead now in a program for the better care of patients rather than to be forced later by the public to follow in such a program."[84]

For the hospital administrators, however, standardization offered the hope of optimizing *their* control over the hospital's increasingly complex structure, through affording the coordination between increasing numbers of professionals, facilitating overview, and getting a better grip on costs. Explicitly comparing medical record-keeping to bookkeeping practices, authors argued that medical records (that are expensive to maintain!) should "cease to be merely factual" and that their "potential value as interpretative documents must be utilized by hospitals":

> There are [currently] no interpretive records. The charts are completed, the case classified on the diagnosis and other indexes. Patient days, admissions and other data are compiled but remain separate records; their relation is seldom shown. . . . We should have a medical report similar in scope to our financial report. We should have a report of our medical services which would enable our staffs as well as the administration to evaluate the medical performance of our institutions.[85]

These different hopes intertwined, clashed, and generated developments that no one can be said to have planned, controlled, or predicted. The motives for the ACS standardizing activities were rather different than the hospital administrators' drives, yet their initiatives intertwined and had consequences that were often paradoxically different from the intentions with which the activities had been set in motion. The record professionals, for example, who themselves emerged as a consequence of the ACS and the administrators' efforts, further refined the layout of preprinted forms to be used as medical records, and thus further stimulated the standardization of individual physicians' tasks.[86] This obviously ran counter to the hope of professional self-determination: here was a group of nonmedically trained people, often women, who were telling physicians how to keep their medical administration![87]

The hospital standardization movement—and in particular the emergence of the patient-centered record—forms a precursor of the contemporary evidence-based medicine movement. Comparing these two movements, we note both the continuity of the ideals of a scientific, effective, and efficient medicine and its change in focus. From an emphasis on the schools that trained physicians, the instruments they employ, and the conditions in which they work, the evidence-based movement now solidly focuses on that which 100 years ago was forbidden terrain: the content of the physician's work. Now physicians are no longer just urged to record clearly what they choose to do: they are now *told* in detail what to do.

Similarly, the drives behind these standardization movements are similar yet distinct. As a century ago, one cannot understand the sudden rise of these movements without taking into account the position in which the medical profession finds itself. Yet whereas 100 years ago, the medical profession was consolidating and enhancing its newly gained status (never a simple nor one-directional endeavor, as this chapter shows), now the medical profession is confronted with new actors challenging its jurisdiction in novel ways. Third-party buyers and patient-consumers have come on the scene, demanding transparency and accountability to an unprecedented degree.

Evidence-based medicine promises this transparency and accountability. Furthermore, evidence-based medicine likewise promises to increase medicine's effectiveness and efficiency. It aims to eradicate unwarranted variation, and wants to see to it that "the highest possible percentage of the best medical knowledge and skill available in a community reaches the patients in the hospitals of that community," as Bottomley phrased it almost 100 years ago.[88]

Standardization is a thoroughly political enterprise in at least two ways. First of all, standardization is political in the sense that the process of standardization is typified by ongoing negotiations between a host of actors, none of whom is in control or oversees all issues that may be at stake.[89] There were many different forces at play in the development of the patient-centered record, with varying motives and interests—and as in most technological development trajectories, the actual course that this technological development took was nonlinear and unpredictable.[90] The development of record-keeping procedures took a different shape in the Netherlands because the Dutch health care network was shaped differently: due to the different position of the Dutch Medical Association, for example, record keeping remained the responsibility of individual physicians and organizations.

Second, standardization is political since it inevitably reorders practices, and such reorderings have consequences that affect the position of actors (through, for example, the distribution of resources and responsibilities). The shifting relations between the health care professions, the disappearance of black hospitals, and the changing legal status of the record in early-twentieth-century U.S. medicine all indicate that it would be a painful mistake to denote standardization as a mere technical issue, not worthy of sociological attention. The position of the patient was affected as well: it is not too exaggerated to state that the introduction of the patient-centered record helped reconfigure the patient in early-twentieth-century U.S. medicine. The creation of the patient-centered record implied an individualization of the poor and the increased valuation of their status as patients through the granting of individual records to them. This increased valuation of the poor at the same time implied a democratization of private patients whose medical information would now be stored in the same files—as one comparable body among many. From "moral minors" whose care was a matter of benevolence or practical necessity (as a means to have access to teaching and research material), and from private patients who were the physician's social peer and employer, a modern patient emerged: a liberal subject endowed with a biomedical body requesting professional care.[91]

2   Standards at Work

A Dynamic Transformation of Medicine

Peter Jansens visits an insurance physician, Dr. Myriam Witts, in Utrecht, the Netherlands. Jansens had parked his car at the town's local dump to fill out some paperwork when a car pulling a trailer drove past him. The trailer had a metal bar sticking out of the back, which sliced through Peter Jansens's door as if it were cardboard and severed his leg above the knee. After Jansens spent a month in the hospital and several weeks on a rehabilitation unit where he had been fitted with a leg brace, Dr. Witts needs to assess Jansens's ability to rejoin the workforce and to determine the level of labor disability. At the end of the visit, after having spoken with Jansens and having read the letters from the treating doctors, she turns to her computer and clicks on the MDC (Medical Disability Criterion) protocol. Clicking through the menus the program offers, and entering bits of text, the protocol automatically creates a comprehensive narrative about Jansens's visit.

John van der Maas, senior resident at the oncology ward of an Academic Hospital in the Netherlands, is doing some paperwork when Karel Gerritsen, a nurse, comes up to him. "John, look here, they messed this up. FRAM-6 [a research protocol for an intensive cancer treatment] says you need this drug dissolved in 500 ml NaCl—and the pharmacy dissolved it in 1,000 ml. What do I do now?" John checks the protocol's drug schedule: "Well . . . I don't think it's too problematic . . . look, if you just give that 1,000 ml of NaCl, he will get the same total amount."

What is it that standards and guidelines do in health care work? What is their impact on the everyday activities of doctors, respiratory therapists, patients, administrators, researchers, and nurses? Popular accounts depict the invasion of standards in health care as a gradual stifling of work practices and the steady depletion of the lifeblood of skills, creativity, and a personalized approach. In an environment with preset rules and regulations, patients become numbers and "interact with impersonal technologies and technicians," and health care workers bemoan the "removal of mystery or excitement" from their work lives.[1] On the other hand, many guideline and information technology enthusiasts promise to "reduce inappropriate variation in services, improve the quality of care, and produce better health outcomes."[2]

In this chapter, we offer an alternative account to stories that either demonize or worship guidelines. Workplaces where standards abound do not look like stifled robot-scapes. They also do not run smoothly like the often invoked metaphor of a well-oiled machine. What becomes crucial to the outcome of standardization processes is the content of the standards and the ways participants designed and implemented the standards. What matters in the encounter between Peter Jansens and Dr. Witts is whether the physician will be able to produce an assessment of Jansens's physical condition and his ability to work that meets legal and scientific requirements, whether she satisfies her immediate supervisor, and whether her report is acceptable to the government agency that will pay out disability benefits. What matters for John van der Maas and Karel Gerritsen is whether patients are satisfied with their enrollment in the research protocols, whether enough patients will enroll so that the protocol will deliver results, whether nurses and physicians are willing to follow the protocol's directions, and whether their participation in this international research project will enhance their careers. Already one can see that Jansens and Witts are not oppressed by the stifling protocols or that the mere presence of a protocol makes internationally collaborative research and disability assessment more effective. Instead, making the protocols work requires the active collaboration of all parties involved.

To get a grasp on the broad theme of standards at work, we confine the discussion to procedural standards, that is, the standards that intervene directly in the organization of work. The chapter consists of two interrelated parts. First, we provide a close reading of the actual tools that constitute a procedural standard. We focus on two procedural standards: a research protocol for the treatment of Hodgkin's disease (FRAM-6), and standardized forms used by insurance physicians to draft their reports of labor disability cases.[3]

Second, we discuss the active role of these standards in work practices, and on their ability to make novel links between work practices, and to transform the skills, capacities, and properties of the work practices involved. Procedural standards, we argue, transform work practices through their coordinating roles: they coordinate work tasks of individuals and of groups within and between work practices. This role, we also point out, is not a self-evident fact. It requires the active and deliberate collaboration of the health care professionals whose work will ultimately be changed.[4] In the conclusion of this chapter, we return to the normative questions raised by the popular accounts we mentioned above, and we illustrate what an alternative politics of standards at work could look like.

The international research protocol and the standardized disability assessment instruments are implicated in different ways in evidence-based medicine. Research protocols are highly detailed prescriptions about what to do when, and in which sequence; the standardized forms are a common means to stimulate complete record keeping and enhance transparency. These tools instantiate different aspects of evidence-based medicine: clinical trials are the sublime arbiter of right versus wrong medicine, and the strictness of these protocols indicates what it means to truly base one's actions upon evidence. Similarly, the standardized reporting forms indicate the way the evidence suggests a certain task should be executed. In addition, standardized tools strive to make physicians' reports more comprehensive, thus allowing other readers to better judge and draw upon the insurance physicians' actions.

We have selected these tools because they represent different branches of standardized medicine, and because they form instances where procedural standards intervene thoroughly in the actual work of those who deal with them. One could argue that thorough impact is actually not typical of many evidence-based clinical practice guidelines: indeed, the fact that many guidelines seem to have little effect on the actual practice of physicians is often lamented[5] (see also Chapter 4). There is a broad spectrum here: many guidelines just end up in piles of unread literature on doctors' desks; other guidelines are read and may partially influence some activities of some care professionals; some guidelines, like the ones discussed here, are collectively implemented. Yet, instead of pondering why some guidelines succeed in changing health care and others do not, this chapter takes up the issue of how any procedural standard is able to affect health care practice. We argue that the active role of procedural standards can arise only if the care professionals themselves interactively take it up: the less they do so, the smaller will be the potential transformative effects of the standards that this chapter will focus on.[6]

Introducing Two Standards: The Research and the Reporting Protocol

International Research Protocol

FRAM-6 was an oncological research protocol for the treatment of patients with Hodgkin's disease who had not adequately responded to ordinary chemotherapeutical treatment. This category of patients generally had a poor prognosis, and this trial was designed to investigate the potential of aggressive, "last hope" treatment. For patients deemed suitable, the protocol prescribed high-dose chemotherapeutical treatment, followed by bone marrow transplantation. The protocol was an international collaborative study, in which nine Dutch and two American centers participated. The thirty-page manuscript started out by discussing the background to the study (the reasons for selecting this disease and these drugs), and summarized the study's objective and its design. After summarizing the known information on the drugs used in the protocol, the patients' eligibility criteria were discussed. To name a few:

• Patients must have histologically proven Hodgkin's disease at diagnosis.
• Patients should have shown resistance to MOPP,[7] as shown by either progression while receiving MOPP or failure to achieve a complete remission after six cycles of MOPP, or relapse within a year of completion of MOPP.
• Patients must have adequate cardiac function (≥ 0.5 ejection fraction), pulmonary function (vital capacity ≥ 70 percent of predicted and a diffusion capacity of ≥ 50 percent), and so forth.

The treatment plan required patients first to receive two courses of cisplatin, cytarabine, and dexamethosone (abbreviated as DHAP), in three- to four-week cycles. If hematological or renal toxicity occurred, the doses had to be reduced, according to included tables (see Table 2.1).

After these cycles, bone marrow from the patient was harvested from (usually) the pelvic bone, and was frozen. Next, the high-dose chemotherapy regimen was outlined (see Table 2.2). The researchers explained the table:

• CYCLOPHOSPHAMIDE: 1.5 g/m2 will be dissolved in 500 cc of D5/W and given over two hours intravenously daily for 4 days (days −6 through −3).

Table 2.1.   Dose Reduction in Case of Renal Toxicity

Serum Creatinine (mg/% µmol/l)	Creatine Clearance (cc/min)	Modification Cisplatin
0.6–1.4 or 50–120	> 60	None
1.5–2.0 or 130–180	40–60	25 percent reduction of CDDP
> 2.0 or > 180	< 40	Delete DDP

Source: FRAM-6 protocol (unpublished work document). The conditions in the first two columns necessitate the change outlined in the last column.

Table 2.2.   The Chemotherapy Regimen

	Day						
	−6	−5	−4	−3	−2	−1	0
BCNU 300 mg/m²	X						
Cyclophosphamide 1.5 g/m²	X	X	X	X			
Etoposide 125 mg/m²	X	X	X				
ABMT							X

Source: FRAM-6 protocol (unpublished work document).

- BCNU:[8] 300 mg/m2 will be dissolved in 100 cc of D5/W and will be given IV piggyback over 30 minutes on day −6 only.
- ETOPOSIDE: will be started on day −6 and given two times/day for three days, each dose being 125 mg/m². Etoposide is dissolved in D5/W NS at a concentration of 1.0 mg/ml and infused intravenously at the rate of 250 mg/hr. To ensure stability of the drug at this concentration, doses greater than 250 mg will be divided into bags of equal

strengths. The pharmacy will mix each bag on call after the completion of the previous dose.

These doses of chemotherapeutic agents are so high that they kill all sensitive cells: cancer cells, hopefully, but also the bone marrow cells, which generate the red blood cells and white blood cells. Without these, one cannot live. This is the essence of bone marrow transplantation: after the high-dose treatment, the bone marrow that was collected is given back to the patient. After a brief period in which the patient is highly sensitive to infection and bleeding, these bone marrow cells should gradually re-create a normal level of red and white blood cells. The protocol specified, therefore, that patients would be admitted to the hospital for the duration of the treatment program. During the period of the high-dose treatment, they would be nursed in a protected room:

> Patients shall be nursed either in the protective environment or in a private room. All patients shall receive oral prophylactic antibiotics starting 10 days prior to [high dose treatment] in order to provide selective decontamination of the gastrointestinal tract. This will be done according to local protocols. Patients shall be discharged from the hospital when the absolute granulocyte count is over 500/mm3 for two consecutive days.

Turning to the second set of protocols, Dutch insurance physicians are responsible for the evaluation of claims of labor disability. These physicians determine whether an individual will be entitled to a disability benefit.[9] Their evaluations, therefore, have both a medical and a legal dimension: they are to fulfill minimum standards of good medical practice, and they have to be legally sound. Their actions may be judged by medical and by legal criteria simultaneously. Disability evaluations may be easy (someone who lost his legs in an accident would unlikely qualify for a position of waiter in a restaurant), but are often very tricky: how much disability does a chronic disease cause? Can marital quarrels lead to psychological dysfunctioning, resulting in labor disability? One of the means devised to help insurance physicians comply with the complicated demands of individual cases and medical and legal requirements are preprinted, standard reporting forms.

Insurance Reporting Standards

Reporting is an important aspect of an insurance physician's work: if a claim evaluation is contested by a client, for example, the report counts as the legal document concerning what has and has not been done. In addition, the quality of the report itself may be taken as an indicator of the quality of the overall work of the insurance physician.

The reporting forms are often developed by the national organizations that employ the insurance physicians (so-called administrative bodies), but sometimes regional offices have their own variations. The insurance physicians use the forms when they report about claim evaluation cases: all they need to do is fill in missing pieces of text, or check the preprinted sentence that they want to use in their report. Often, the preset forms (also referred to as the "reporting protocol") are available as a software package: all the physician has to do is to click on the prewritten sentences to select (or delete) them. Almost all forms are ordered by the headings "problem," "investigation," "discussion," "conclusion," and "plan." Each heading is followed by standard phrases. In some cases, this means that the physician only has to fill in the blanks, as in the following example:

Possibilities and limitations:

The limitations started _____, because _____

The task capacity has also been registered using the Form Function Information System to allow automated processing of this information. In this form, the task capacity is graded, if necessary with an explanation. For a more detailed registration of the client's task capacity, see the verbal description of the task capacity profile that follows the labor expert's investigation.

In this case, the last paragraph of this subheading is ready-made, and will thus appear in every report. It refers the reader to two other documents: an electronic form, reporting the elaborate investigation of the mental and physical capacities of the client that is standard procedure in all claim evaluations, and a more detailed, final evaluation document that is made after the client is seen by the labor expert. The physician only needs to fill in the missing data in the first sentence. In most cases, however, the physician can choose from an elaborate menu of sentences. A different form had the following options under the subheading "possibilities and limitations" (only five out of a total of nine options are listed here):

Possibilities and limitations:

The possibilities with regards to the most relevant task capacity items are as follows: _____

The possibilities and limitations of the client has also been registered using the Form Function Information System to allow automated processing of this information. In this form, the task capacity is graded, if necessary with an explanation. For a more detailed registration of the client's task capacity, see the verbal description of the task capacity profile that follows the labor expert's investigation.

So much information about the health condition of the client is missing, that not even a preliminary judgment about the possibilities to function can be given. More information has to be gathered first. When this information has been received, an additional report will be made.

The possibilities and limitations of the client have not changed since the last evaluation at _____

The health condition of the client implies, for a longer period of time, a severely limited possibility to function which is clearly not compatible with paid labor. This is due especially to the fact that the client is

admitted to a _____

bedridden

incapable to function personally or socially

The possibilities of the client have decreased since the last evaluation but this is largely due to a different disease-cause

In this example, the physicians can select from several prewritten phrases. Depending on the option chosen, they have to fill in a blank, or (in the case of the fourth option listed here), to make a further selection.

Similarly, the conclusions to the claim evaluations are often standard phrases. In one office, the insurance physician had to merely fill in and cross out several small pieces of text (the following text is only one of the texts that can be selected under the heading "discussion and conclusion"):

Client is a _____ year old _____, who has since _____ failed to do his/her job completely/partially, because _____

Considering the information obtained through anamnesis and our investigation, and considering the content of the information put at our disposal from the curative sector, the following is justified:

The current insurance medical investigation shows a condition that may change significantly within 3 months because the client is in a recovery phase / after a surgical intervention / after a _____

The determination of a task capacity profile, therefore, is not (yet) called for.

The client's task capacity is limited as a directly and objectively determinable medical consequence of a disease and/or infirmity

For the remaining task capacity related to the ability to work see the more detailed and quantified verbal registration of the task capacity profile.

STANDARDS AS COORDINATING DEVICES

The insurance reporting forms and the oncology research protocol are very different devices. The former focuses only on the reporting of professional work, while the latter outlines a whole diagnostic and therapeutic trajectory. Also, the disability insurance reporting forms were all made in-house, and could differ per regional office, while FRAM-6 was an internationally developed protocol whose main point was to render the testing of this particular drug regime uniform throughout all the participating sites. The forms' scope also differed. The reporting form addressed the work of the individual insurance physician. The oncological protocol, in contrast, addressed and affected oncologists, patients, nurses, and pharmacies alike.

But the important similarity is that both forms standardize a set of practices, actors, and situations. They intervene in a specified situation and prescribe a set of activities that should be performed in a similar way in order to achieve results comparable over time and space. According to the designers of the form, it should not matter whether a plumber or a business executive presented with disability complaints to a doctor, whether the examination occurred in Utrecht or in Eijsden, whether the evaluation was simple or contested, and what the patient's current physical situation is. What matters is that the insurance physician fills in each form in an identical manner, using the same phrases in the same sequence. Similarly, once a patient fulfills the FRAM-6 criteria and is included in the study, the protocol designers and people interpreting the results obtained from the study assume that the protocol follows its precharted course.

What, then, is it that these tools do? *Both tools coordinate—and thereby transform—the activities of the individuals who work with them.* They *structure* and *sequence* these activities: checking off the sentences or actions to undertake. The protocols give shape to and order the activities of the health care worker in a prespecified way. The standards mediate the health care worker's tasks by delegating the exact sequence in which tasks need to be performed and the overall structure of work tasks.[10] In these standards, a preferred organization of steps to take and sentences to use is already embedded, and by drawing upon them, health care workers automatically integrate this organization into their activities—without having to perform this organizing work themselves.

Because of this partial delegation of tasks from worker to tool, the procedural standards afford an increase in the overall complexity of health care providers' work. When drawing upon the research protocol, doctors and nurses could handle the highly complex therapeutic treatment modalities of FRAM-6: over a short time period, several cycles of combined, highly toxic drugs were given, through varying routes and in varying doses. Likewise, the reporting forms facilitate the reporting task of the insurance physicians: by simply following the headings and preprinted phrases on the form, their task is limited to filling in the missing pieces. The task of integrating the overall report, of not overlooking headings, and of ensuring a structure that meets professional and legal requirements is delegated to the form. Streamlining the individual steps leads to an increase of the complexity of the overall task without a concurrent increase of complexity of the individual steps.

Through structuring and sequencing an individual's tasks, in addition, the medical content of these tasks changes. It is obvious that by checking the patient's eligibility criteria, and by mixing and administering the drugs according to the precisely outlined tables in the protocol, the health care professional is administering a novel therapy designed by international experts at the front lines of oncological research. Less obviously, the reporting form similarly affects the content of the work performed. Although aimed at the (post hoc) reporting of a clinical procedure, this insurance reporting standard nevertheless affects that procedure as well. Consider the following reporting form, which uses a phrase (under the heading "discussion") designed to outline situations in which the health of a client is incompatible with performing work. These cases need to be clearly circumscribed because they lead to a 100 percent labor disability evaluation without requiring the standard, time-consuming (and taxing) evaluation of the mental and physical capacities of the client. The phrase contains four options to select, of which one needs further specification (see above):

The health condition of the client implies, for a longer period of time, a severely limited possibility to function which is clearly not compatible with paid labor. This is due especially to the fact that the client is

admitted to a _____

bedridden

incapable to function personally or socially

The reporting form of a different office has a similar phrase, also under the heading "discussion." In this form, the "inability to function personally and socially" is split up into further specifications:

This inability is demonstrated in the disturbance that occurred in the functioning regarding the care of self, family relations and social contacts outside of the family (including maintaining work relations, if any). The functioning of the client in these roles is currently as follows:

Care of self: _____

Family relations: _____

Social contacts outside the family: _____

When using this form physicians cannot merely check the option "inability to function personally and socially." They will have to further specify and legitimate this evaluation by explicating just what this inability consists of.

A different form from a third office asks the insurance physician to describe the social and personal functioning under the heading "investigation," specified in three "roles" (care of self, family relations, social contacts outside the family). In this case, the physician is prompted to include these roles in every evaluation, even when there is no question of an evident inability to work.

Different insurance physicians will have their evaluations organized in varying ways, depending on the form they employ. The forms affect what is and what is not discussed, when, and in how much detail. Such an organization and resulting discussion matters because the forms may yield subtle differences between the evaluation of cases in various locales. When personal and social functioning is given a prominent place on the reporting form, this consideration might play a more central role in the overall claim evaluation. It will first prompt physicians to be more exhaustive in their questioning on these matters, and then also steer their conclusions *because* these issues are so prominent.[11]

In these examples, we stressed how the coordinating activities of the procedural standards affect the tasks of the individual health care worker—with regards to both their complexity and their content. Through coordinating these individuals' activities the standards also carve out and coordinate larger configurations of individuals and tools. When insurance physicians draw upon a standardized reporting form, they automatically use formulations that have been carefully crafted in accordance with the Dutch Disability Act and its interpretation in court. The phrases mentioned above are riddled with references to laws. The detailed phrasing about the interactions with the labor expert and the task capacity profile and the remark that "the client's task capacity is limited as a directly and objectively determinable medical consequence of a disease and/or infirmity" are directly derived from the Disability Act. Likewise, clicking on the phrase that the "possibilities have decreased since the last evaluation but this is largely due to a different disease-cause" invokes a law that regulates cases due to "similar causes," and creates a report that clearly orients itself to this law.

In addition, using the insurance reporting protocol creates scientifically structured reports: the headings follow the pattern of a hypothetical-deductive scientific evaluation of a claim (from problem to investigation to discussion to plan). No matter how messy or eclectic the individual steps and the lines of reasoning were, in their post hoc description, they all end up in their proper place. Once written down, the temporal pattern of the original claim evaluation is lost; all that remains is the "true description," which depicts a logical, stepwise, and orderly evaluation of a claim.[12]

In these ways, the reports produced follow a standard layout, fusing the legal framework within which insurance medicine operates with positivist, scientific notions of a proper investigation, based on available evidence that follows epidemiological principles. Further, the reporting forms force the insurance physicians to describe and legitimate their activities in detail: headings and blanks that are not filled in stand out and suggest incompleteness. In unstructured forms, physicians might summarize a claim evaluation in a few sentences. Yet when there are separate headings for "problem," "investigation," and "discussion," the physicians will at least have to disentangle their considerations and actions into parts that fit these respective categories. These elaborations, which are themselves ordered according to the scientific logic of the reporting form, further strengthen its legal and scientific credibility.

As an additional effect, the uniformity and clarity that these reporting forms were supposed to bring to the final reports would make it easier for colleagues and other parties (clients, controlling physicians, maybe judges) to use the reports for their purposes. Because every report will be structured in a similar way and with sufficient depth, third parties would know what type of form to expect, would know where to find certain information, and would be able to actually understand and use that information.

Finally, the reporting protocol embeds several other guidelines that the National Institute for Social Insurance has issued (see Chapter 4 for a detailed discussion of these guidelines). For example, the way the "inability to function personally and socially" is defined in three roles in the forms discussed above is directly drawn from a guideline that discusses when a client can be declared fully unfit for labor without having to investigate precisely the mental and physical capabilities of the client. By filling in the form, the physician is automatically integrated into the paths these guidelines draw—and thereby into all the specific legal and medical professional articulations that these guidelines make.

While coordinating individual insurance physicians' activities, the protocols align work practices with the legal requirements stated in the law and refined in court discussions about contested cases; with medical-professional discussions about the validity of certain inferences in the evaluation of disability; with the aims of the insurance physicians' profession to reduce practice variations and make its work more evidence-based; and with the demands of third parties and politicians worried about the high number of disability cases. Although insurance physicians in the Utrecht office might be merely pondering the complexities of an individual client when they fill in the form, the simple act of drawing upon this procedural standard renders their activities similar to those of their colleagues spread throughout the country.

Likewise, the FRAM-6 research protocol also ties the activities of the individuals working with it into larger wholes. The standard brings together different professionals around one case: it articulates the activities of nurses, oncologists, pharmacists, and cardiologists (e.g., planning the isolation rooms, checking toxicity levels, mixing the drug "cocktails," and measuring the cardiac ejection fraction). As in the case of the individual insurance physician, the complexity of this collective arrangement is made doable by the standard.[13] It outlines the distribution and content of tasks, and ensures that the individual activities of all those involved become an integral part of the larger care process. Because of the standard, doctors, nurses, and pharmacists know how their work tasks interrelate and where patients are in their therapeutic trajectories. Its checklists and tables afford the linking of actions and events over different sites and times without face-to-face interaction between the doctors and nurses, and without doctors having to personally check when and how a drug has been given.[14]

More prominently than in the case of the reporting standard, the research protocol also feeds into the construction of novel communities.[15] The insurance reporting standard was written by insurance physicians for insurance physicians; although it is part of the ongoing process of defining and innovating the profession, it does not completely redraw its professional borders. Research protocols, however, turn the patient into an entry of a randomized clinical research trial, and the doctors into internationally collaborating, innovative clinical scientists.[16] Interrelated series of research protocols form the material core that organizes large, internationally distributed, and closely knit communities of oncologists.[17] The patient becomes part of an experimental or a control group, and the international collaboration distinguishes those clinicians who generate the evidence from those who are merely expected to change their working practices accordingly.

In sum, allowing the sequence and content of their actions to be standardized and delegating part of the control over their work to the procedural standard enrolls these individuals in larger networks. In this movement, the work transcends the boundaries of the local work sites, and becomes attached to a plethora of specific concerns, developments, drives, and communities that defines their professional field and its social and political environment. Their own trajectories, in other words, become transformed and linked to other trajectories—the pasts, presents, and possible futures of other researchers, physicians, patients, novel drugs, the evidence-based movement, social security laws, and so forth.

It is important to stress that these standards are *active* tools, doing part of the coordination that interrelates work practices and keeps them going. In their study of technical design standards, Schmidt and Werle state that such standards "specify the relational properties of individual technical components that are necessary for the overall system to achieve its technical functionality."[18] By conforming to the same set of standards outlining the "handshake protocol,"[19] error-handling, coding schemes, and so forth, for example, compatibility between fax machines of different manufacturers used all over the globe is guaranteed. Likewise, the procedural standards discussed here specify the relationships between health care professionals and other actors necessary for functional cancer treatment. Schmidt and Werle, however, argue that standards facilitate "coordination among the actors involved in a technical system," and their book discusses the "considerable coordinative endeavor" of the process of standard setting.[20] Although we agree with the latter observation,[21] we would rather emphasize how standards *actively* coordinate work tasks rather than facilitate their coordination. Procedural standards' power to transform tasks and work practices lies in the ongoing delegation of coordinative tasks. Following Edwin Hutchins, we see procedural standards as acting *with* health care professionals in the performance of this new task. The protocols are not tools that human actors draw upon to facilitate their work; they are not tools that stand "between the user and the task."[22] They operate in conjunction with the human actors, performing a task that neither the protocol nor the health care professional could perform alone. The insurance physicians, oncologists, and nurses interact with the protocols rather than merely appropriating the protocols at will. The latter formulation implies an absolute distribution of agency—all to the health care professionals, none to the artifact—which does not do justice to the constitutive role of the standard in the work task, nor to the lack of latitude of the health care professional in shaping the task.

PROCEDURAL STANDARDS IN PRACTICE

Discussions of introducing and using standards and guidelines in medicine abound with images of domination and oppression. Critics argue that guidelines render physicians' skills superfluous when the tools determine paths of action. Physicians would merely have to understand directions and do what they are told; they would certainly not be expected to think for themselves. The doctor would be reduced "to a mindless cook."[23] Discussing resuscitation guidelines, the American Heart Association literally warned: "The team leader must be ever observant. Though the algorithms provide a good 'cookbook,' the team leader must remain a 'thinking cook.' "[24] In short, guidelines can become a form of "tyrannical domination" against which physicians' discretion should be protected.[25] Standardization, in this view, is on a par with domination and oppression: standardization implies unequivocally subjecting the involved actors' activities to the network builders', that is, the guideline designers', goals.[26]

We indicated in the previous chapter how standards are the result of historically situated, distributed work of a multitude of actors. In this chapter, we draw attention to the fact that health care providers actively and deliberately try to make the guidelines work for them; their orientation toward guidelines is pragmatic. If they follow the standard's directions it is because they consider it useful for the tasks at hand. And if they do not, the guideline likely did not match the requirements of their daily work practices, or they did not consider the benefits gained from aligning themselves with the guideline worth the cost of the exigencies posed by this alignment. In observing the utilization of procedural guidelines in medical practices, it is striking that patients and medical personnel are *not* turned into mindless followers of some preset recipe. From their perspectives, the guideline is drawn upon to advance their own goals and professional trajectories. For all those involved, the guideline is not a goal in itself but a *means*, acted upon in terms of their own aims and the local constraints structuring the situation in which the guideline happens to be placed.[27]

For the insurance physician, for example, the reporting protocol is first and foremost a practical tool to speed up the reporting process while producing state-of-the-art reports. Physicians' conformity to the protocol can in no way be construed as mere docility: they draw upon the protocol because it appears to cultivate their purpose more than it impedes it. Moreover, the insurance reporting protocols leave room for individual elaboration. Two physicians explain:

> Everybody adapts them, more or less, to their own insights. It is being used as framework. That's what it looks like—and you can move things here or add things there . . . as I did. . . . The social history wasn't listed at all, so I made a heading for that. (IE)

> Some have just a list of the required main headings, and others have created ten or more detailed subheadings for themselves in every category. Both are OK, individual elaboration is allowed, as long as the framework of the standard remains unaffected. (DC)

Some local offices have adapted their administrative body's national reporting protocol, and sometimes individual insurance physicians continue to appropriate these protocols. As long as these adaptations and
added details remain within the framework of the office's reporting protocol, insurance physicians can construe their own reporting protocols
to match their particular working style.

Patients bring their own goals and hopes to the research protocol.
Viewed from the trajectory of patients, a protocol such as FRAM-6 is a
source of hope, often the only perceived means to combat the disease
that has stricken them. For many patients enrolled in FRAM-6, the research protocol is the last Western medical therapy possible with (albeit
little) chance of cure. They rarely care about the research goals of the
protocol (although sometimes they do); all they care about is preserving life and having a possible future. Drawing upon the protocol in this
way, patients will often negotiate their eligibility for a protocol, try to
adjust the times of the chemotherapy courses to their convenience, or
skip courses when they no longer see a meaningful link between their
own future and the protocol's trajectory. Similarly, some protocols require patients to register the amount of fluids or food they take in, or the
quantities of urine they produce. Here as well, patients are sometimes
little motivated to fulfill these chores, which they often see as superfluous. Yet, the doctrine of informed consent makes their willingness to
take on the grueling demands of the protocol an informed, if not explicit
choice.[28] Similarly for patients with disabilities, the insurance recording
protocol might mean a validation of their physical limitations and mental anguish. The organization of the protocol and the evaluation of their
status charts a possible future. The protocol prescribes the limits and
possibilities of monetary reimbursement and physical activity.

In their turn, many health care workers evaluate FRAM-6 and similar research protocols in light of their personal research interests. A major reason why oncologists go through all the trouble of discussing and
implementing the protocol criteria and drug schedules is that their careers are tied up with publishing research results. Also, the protocol affords them, and the institution in which they work, status, new patients,
and greater financial latitude. Protocols allow nurses contact with new
drugs, with new possibilities for cure, with a wider variety of patients
and treatment plans, and with the status and career opportunities that
come with clinical research work in highly specialized fields.

The following example underscores how the protocol becomes integrated in patient and staff trajectories:

> In a regional oncology meeting, Grafson is discussed, a young man suffering from Hodgkin's disease. He has had an early relapse after MOPP treatment, and the bone scan shows several infiltrations in his skeleton. The question from the oncologist of a nearby hospital is whether this patient would be eligible for FRAM-6, in which case he can refer him to the regional university hospital. The discussion centers around whether bone infiltrations preclude bone marrow transplantation: the bone marrow could then itself contain tumorous cells, which would be reinfused *after* the high-dose therapy. The protocol, however, does not exclude such patients: it merely demands that the bone marrow, upon testing, is "clean." Still, the physicians doubt whether they want to take this risk. "It's safety first," one of them remarks. "We can also use one of his family members as a bone marrow donor." This, however, is a less established approach in these types of patients—and FRAM-6 would not apply. "And if we go outside of FRAM-6," the oncologist continues, "we can think whether we know any better drugs than DHAP. We're out of the protocol now anyway."

For the physicians discussing Grafson, FRAM-6 was one of the possible things they could do for this patient. Patient interests, here, are primary. Rather than searching for the right patients for the protocol,[29] oncologists often *search the right protocol for their patients*. FRAM-6 did not exclude Grafson, but the physicians chose not to enroll him. Similarly, protocols are sometimes primarily a means to obtain drugs free of charge (in the case of industry-subsidized trials, for example), or a place where a patient can be sent for whom there is really nothing more to do so that the final verdict can be delayed.

To achieve the aim of being part of a research team, of receiving last-hope therapy, or of training a state-of-the-art insurance physician, everyone involved has to submit to the procedural standard. They have to allow the delegation of responsibilities to the tool for it to function. They have to truly hand over some of the control over their actions to the standard for it to coordinate their activities and articulate them to others.

This submission, however, does not imply a domination of the health care worker by the protocol. The notion of submission, rather, points to the fact that health care workers actively allow themselves to be affected by the procedural standard. A protocol, after all, only does something when it is picked up, interpreted, acted upon, and passed on. Only when physicians and families act upon FRAM-6's guidelines can the protocol transform the work of oncologists and patients' chances. The reverse is also true: health care workers become involved in the activity of doing research only when they handle, read, mark, check, and pass on research protocols.

Rather than a *passive* act of being disempowered, we want to construe the activity of working with standards as an *active act of allowing oneself to be transformed while at the same time transforming the standard*.[30] A first, basic sense in which this is the case is that for those involved to commit themselves to the guideline, they have to be given some leeway or discretion to adapt the guideline. Total control of physicians' activities is impossible in current medical practice; they would simply not cooperate. Oncologists would sabotage the protocol by not entering patients; insurance physicians could resist overly detailed reporting protocols by systematically deleting the preset phrases, or using a less prestructured heading to enter the information in the way they deem important. For oncological nurses, similarly, attempting total control can lead to subtle sabotage. By working to the rule, nurses can create total chaos, or by informing patients in the right way, they can ensure that no patient gives permission for a certain research protocol to be used on her or him.[31] As ethnomethodological texts have repeatedly shown, full control in specifications is impossible.[32] Even if one stipulates in 347 pages how two workers need to change a light bulb in a nuclear plant,[33] the guidelines simply cannot capture the full extent of the requisite work in the finest detail. All such attempts are necessarily at once overdetermined and continually indeterminate.

More important, however, working with guidelines is an active act because of the required proficiency. Rather than a matter for "mindless cooks," active submission appears to be a highly skillful activity. Over time, nurses and doctors form what Knorr-Cetina has called a "common lifeworld" with these procedural standards.[34] A kind of embodied expertise emerges in unison with the guidelines' activities: the nurses know where to find the medication tables at a glance, and they learn to discriminate between the medical events that are relevant for the progression of the tool.[35] This expertise is a necessary condition for the guideline's functioning. Continually, unforeseen contingencies occur, threatening the guideline's path; continually, nurses or physicians have to take ad hoc measures to keep the guideline functioning, as we saw in the at the beginning of this chapter, where Karel Gerritsen was confronted with a wrongly dissolved chemotherapeutic drug.

Dispensaries dissolve drugs erroneously, doctors' mistakes have to be corrected by nurses—the list of adjustments is endless. A sudden drop in the white blood cell count can require ad hoc intervention to keep the patient's trajectory linked to the protocol. Here, a nurse working in the oncological ward points at the expertise involved in making research protocols work with patients, families, and residents, and getting to know a new protocol:

> Look, all those protocols. It's interesting stuff. But they [the physicians] tend to just dump these things on us. I mean, they tell us we're such a great ward, so capable and all that. But then they just hand us the protocol and tell us that "they'll hear from us when there is a problem." They don't realize the extra work it takes, the extra time you have to spend with family. And if it is a new protocol, and they don't give us the details, what *can* we tell the family? How sick are they going to be? When? If they don't tell us, if we don't *know* how these protocols tick, we're at a loss when we've got to inform them. Also, you get more insecure when, say, a fever develops. If you know the protocol, you know, for instance, that a brief fever at time X is nothing to worry about. That you don't need to do a blood culture (which you're supposed to according to our in-house protocols), since that will be lots of wasted work for nothing. And even if there is an inexperienced resident, who is unsure about this fever, we can still steer them in the right direction. That's no problem. They ask us for the right dosages for medication all the time. But if you don't *know* the protocol, again, we also do not know what to expect—and you end up doing more blood cultures, harassing the patient sometimes four times a day, doing more X rays, and so forth.

The nurse points to the time needed to acquire skills and proficiencies—and of the problems that may ensue when this does not happen. The skillful interactions of health care workers with the protocol is a *prerequisite* for its functioning: it is what affords the tool to transform concurrently their working lives and the lives of their patients.

Insurance physicians, likewise, become highly skilled in dealing with their reporting protocols. They refer to their abbreviation libraries with which they build up reports, and the automated "claim-clicks" through which prefabricated sentences are put together with a few clicks of the mouse. They learn to produce several-page reports within a few seconds. In addition, they become experts in predicting the effect of the reports they create. They know that certain phrases are easier to counteract when a case is contested. Likewise, they know how to write someone "in" and "out" a disability benefit. Referring to the possibility of declaring someone "fully unfit for labor" by stressing his or her "inability to function personally and socially," the following insurance physician describes what he called a typical case:

> If someone functions reasonably well, personally and socially, but you know that she's on the edge, she can still keep her house in order—when you're talking about a woman who, normally speaking, also does part of the housekeeping . . . Say she has always worked, yet she has stopped because she was no longer psychologically able to keep doing her work; her children and husband help out. When you would then say: "OK, get back to work," then you can predict that she'll not pull that off, psychologically. According to the rules, she should be fit for work, but . . . So I pick the phrase in the protocol that says "I expect a clear deterioration soon." You build a story: if by determining her capacities, and by sending her back to work you'd cause a psychological decompensation, then you can avoid that by steering towards that phrase. (RC)

By depicting this case in a specific way (by emphasizing the expected deterioration of the situation rather than the fact that the person is "able to function personally and socially"), the insurance physician creates a reporting form that will easily pass the eyes of critical beholders: this has become a clear case of being "fully unfit for labor."[36]

In addition, the insurance physicians using the reporting protocol faced an interesting development that threatened to undo much of the initial reasons that were behind the introduction of the reporting protocol. Physicians reported in interviews that creating standard and elaborate narratives actually reduced the usability and the transparency of the final reports. The physicians explained:

> I use my own version. . . . There are so many standard phrases in the ordinary reports, I don't think that's good . . . you have to look for the usable information. . . . Many others use the claim-click and then you often see a discussion with standard phrases, one or two added phrases, and then more standard phrases. You then have to really search what the considerations were. . . . In my discussion the text is mine, it doesn't come from the computer, I make it up myself. . . . Everyone should do that. If you have so much standard text, it become too easy to just push that button and add some more. (DE)

> Many others add many standard things, but I keep it relatively unstructured. . . . I think that if you don't do that, you will start to forget what you're actually writing down. You're just clicking, filling in the blanks.

> By keeping it unstructured you force yourself constantly to think about what you write and not to say, well, this is about backs so let me call up and enter the piece we have about backs. (IE)

> You'll have to write the largest part yourself. You can standardize only so much, since otherwise you get an empty report with only standard phrases that could be true for anyone. (NC)

Too many standard phrases, these physicians argued, actually decreased the readability and information value of the reports. Rather than enabling a smooth articulation to the expectations of colleagues and supervising physicians, the reporting protocols might yield "empty reports" and hinder a smooth and fast use of the reports. The similarity of the phrases, and the impossibility of judging whether a sentence is entered as a standard "click" or a result of a thoughtful weighing of words threatens to obscure the transparency that the protocol attempted to introduce. To avoid this possibility, the insurance physicians again skillfully have to judge when standard phrases become too much, and how to find a balance between entering unstructured text and drawing upon standard prose to create a readable yet legally and professionally viable report.

We do not point at these instances of "standards-tinkering" to demonstrate the resistance of actors to domination. Rather, these instances illustrate how health care workers have become experts in handling, dealing with, and being affected by the standard. This newly developed expertise makes the artifact's functioning possible. Working with standards does not imply that staff members' activities become more machinelike or mechanized. This might be counterintuitive because the popular public image associates standardization with an oppressive, tightly circumscribed performance of human tasks.[37] Rather, we have observed highly skillful and creative activities in the interactions with standards. Moreover, aggregate and more complex institutional configurations might emerge through the interactions of the individually standardized activities: top-level research, for example, or the fast, uniform, and readable production of reports.[38]

The standards and health care providers, then, mutually transform each other during their interactions. The therapeutic skills nurses acquire because they submit to the requirements of the standards generate innovative collective work practices irreducible to either humans or protocols alone. Because nurses and physicians skillfully appropriate the tool for their own purposes, the procedural standard is able to structure and sequence their activities. The skills of the health care workers making the standard work and the standard's corresponding effect on their work are intrinsically intertwined. Often studies of procedural standards at work highlight the need for human skills to work around the limits of such tools. Health care providers are supposed to fill in the gap between the intricate, fluid nature of work practices and the preset, formal functioning of standardizing tools.[39] Such a focus, however, overlooks how work skills are not aimed at undoing limits or problems, but at allowing the tool's transformation of the workplace.[40]

IS STANDARDIZATION WORTH THE EFFORT?

In this chapter, we have discussed procedural standards as *coordinating devices*, structuring and sequencing the practice of those individuals that work with them. Because of their active, coordinating functions, protocols afford an increase in the overall complexity of the work of health care professionals, and they transform the medical content of this work. The result is a *standardized work practice*. In addition, while coordinating the activities of individuals, the standards carve out and coordinate larger collectives to which these individuals become associated. Procedural standards form an important part of the glue that ties high-powered research oncologists, severely ill patients, and specialized research nurses together, and that articulate their activities with one another and with the legal, professional, political, and managerial pressures that they face.[41] Tools as described here are as crucially involved in generating the evidence as well as in distributing it—and in both cases, what counts as evidence is partially determined by the nature of the tool and the transformations it undergoes in its diffusion.[42]

This power of procedural standards to create new configurations depends on changes in the work activities of those who interact with these standards. In order for coordinating tools to function, data entry and output interpretation need to be done with a certain level of precision and adherence to guidelines. This implies a standardization of certain of these workers' activities: they can only expect the proper coordinating functioning of a guideline if they themselves act in accordance with its demands.

The active roles of standards, however, does not imply a subordination of health care workers, turning them into "judgmental dopes"—passive, mindless followers of rigid protocols.[43] Standardized work practices do not require a mechanical sequencing of health care workers' activities. Procedural standards are inevitably appropriated by the actors handling them: patients desiring the treatment the protocol affords, and oncologists and nurses focusing on the care for their patients and the research opportunities that the protocol offers. Health care workers have to *submit actively* to these standards' demands to fulfill these promises. They have to forego a position of full control or self-determination and let themselves be acted upon. The result is a practice in which health care workers act *with* the standard: they act skillfully to match the standard to the actual demands of ongoing work, to keep the standard functioning, and, in doing so, to allow their own work to be transformed through the standard's coordinating activity.[44]

What does this analysis mean for a more normative appraisal of standards and the standardization of work practices? The popular accounts that we started out with at the beginning of this chapter yield a clear-cut political position vis-à-vis standardization. The introduction of more and more guidelines, prefixed checklists, and other tools that impose a preset format on the work activities of health care workers would be deemed either a great loss of creative intelligence or a great gain in efficiency and rationality. The moral of those stories is that a practice's worth lies either in the inherent rationality of the standards (thus abating the health care workers' irrationalities) or in the health care worker's skills and clinical judgment (which the standards subsequently threaten). In this analysis, we have attempted to undo this either/or mode of argumentation. We have argued, alternatively, that the generative power of procedural standards *thrives* on the local expertise the nurses and doctors develop in their interaction with these tools—and vice versa. Standardization does not result in an obedient workforce, with individual health care workers accomplishing their tasks in a rigid, preprogrammed fashion. Quite the contrary: affording skillful and nonpredetermined interactions with the procedural standards enhances their generative power. A proper (both effective and desirable) deployment of procedural standards creates a synergy between the staff members' embodied expertise and the tool's coordinating activity, in which expertise and coordination mutually reinforce each other. The more local expertise emerges and is deployed, the more the standard is afforded to transform the practice into the most intricate details.[45]

The normative question becomes what the *specific* transformations are that a standard brings to the practice of which it becomes a part. Bluntly put, the ultimate question becomes whether the standardization achieved is worth the active submission of health care workers. Does the loss of self-control that comes with the delegation of coordinating activities to the standard yield enough returns? The relevant questions to be asked become *which* geographies and architectures the standards help to emerge, *how* they transform the work tasks of health care workers, *how* this subsequently affects the position of staff members, patients, managers, and other involved actors, and how the investments and benefits of the new configuration are distributed. Different configurations of staff members and procedural standards produce very different answers to these questions. In the following chapter, for example, we show that at this moment, for most health care professionals, this question is apparently answered negatively, since they cannot be said to submit actively to the requirements of the increased influx of clinical practice guidelines.

Our conceptualization of standardization at work implies two important points leading to a particular view on the politics of standardization in the workplace. First, the question about the benefits and harms of standardization can be answered only on a case-by-case basis: specific standards may distribute benefits in very different ways. The benefits involved can vary highly, and will be different for the different groups involved. Although in this chapter we have mainly looked at benefits in terms of enhancing the skills and capacities of health care workers, benefits should be taken broadly, including greater decision power, financial remuneration, increased prestige, greater quality of the work (for both patients and health care workers), and emotional satisfaction. Second, the benefits of a specific standard may not be evenly distributed throughout the practice. Some groups may benefit more than others. Yet, in order for standardization to be successful, this distribution of benefits should be closely monitored.

In some cases, for example, standards are implemented mostly for the sake of standardization itself and benefits are difficult to detect for the people implementing the standards. In line with a prevalent managerial drive to control and oversee the work of professionals, standards

are introduced to erase fluid work patterns and replace them with protocolized, rigidly defined sequences of tasks for the single purpose of
rationalizing the practice. In such situations, there is no clear-cut benefit emerging anywhere from the alignment of staff members with the
standard: the only benefit, often only perceived by management, lies in
the alignment itself. The standards do not allow the emergence of new
tasks, nor the import of relevant new evidence, but reroute and reify
already existing ones. The result is that in a misplaced equation of standardization with quality—whether of the care delivered or of the staff
members' work—uniformity is introduced for uniformity's sake.[46]

The case of the FRAM-6 research protocol shows how a standard
might bring much to a practice and to those whose lives are tied up
with it—but it is equally a clear example of the difficulties involved in
attempting to weigh the costs and benefits. For the oncologists, the cost-
benefit ratio seems to favor the benefit side. Their active submission to
the protocol's instructions yields immediate returns for their research
careers, their status vis-à-vis other oncological practices, and their capacity to offer hope to very ill patients. Nurses likewise become enrolled in research practices and high-status medical domains. In their
case, however, the evaluation is less straightforward. Their careers are
less directly tied up with oncological research: although their work is
strongly affected by the coming of research protocols, their names appear only rarely on the publications that come out of these trials.[47] They
are often caught between the severe demands of the protocols and the
patients' attempt to negotiate shortcuts and exceptions—and when they
do not know the underlying logic of the protocol, they are in no position to articulate smoothly all these demands. Finally, in terms of the
patients themselves, although they are at the heart of the protocol, and
although their fate is tied up with the standard in a way incomparable
to any other involved actor, their benefit is the most unclear of all. For
some, being offered a last straw of hope of even living a few months
longer is in and of itself infinitely more important than all the pain and
regulations to which they will have to submit. For others, however, the
offer of a last try might be too hard to resist, although they might have
been served better by a much more peaceful, albeit maybe somewhat
shorter, end of their lives.

The insurance physicians' reporting protocol, finally, helps them perform their work according to the political, professional, and legal pres-

sures that typify their working environment. In this case, the interesting question becomes whether the transparency that the tool attempts to bring to their work will not be obstructed by the tendency to further refine preset phrases in the protocol. In other words, the issue at stake is to find the optimal interaction level between standard and health care worker. Too much detail in the standard seems to make void the benefits of standardization. As is often the case, the crucial and difficult question is at which points and until what lengths standardization benefits whom and how. The question, we hope to have shown, has no easy answers—although both critics and advocates believe otherwise. In the following chapter, we take such a cost-benefit analysis to a macro level and investigate how the medical professions as a whole react to the recent influx of clinical practice guidelines.

3   From Autonomy to Accountability?

Clinical Practice Guidelines and Professionalization

CLINICAL PRACTICE GUIDELINES

Some of the "most successful"[1] and "widely accepted"[2] clinical practice guidelines are the CPR and ACLS protocols that detail the steps to be undertaken when someone suffers a cardiac arrest. About every eight years, the American Heart Association organizes a major conference to update these protocols. At the conference different expert groups go over the accumulated evidence, discuss clinical and ethical aspects of first aid life-saving, and formulate recommendations. When approved, these recommendations are translated into protocol changes and incorporated into training programs. Although even CPR protocols function far from perfectly,[3] they approach the best of what clinical guidelines have to offer. Backed up with scientific evidence and powerful organizations, they encourage widespread consistency in a situation where optimally effective intervention seems highly warranted. Hospitals in the United States now have an interdisciplinary "code" team that performs similar actions when faced with a cardiac arrest. Outside the hospital, CPR forms the organizing principle for a community approach to first aid. Under ideal circumstances, people who would otherwise have died a sudden death might be stabilized in the hospital. From a professional point of view, CPR protocols render the dying process securely under medical jurisdiction (instead of, for example, under the realm of religion) and preserve a clear medical hierarchy of first aid responders, emergency medical technicians (EMTs), paramedics, and a team approach in the emergency department. As can be readily seen from professional publications, paramedics and emergency staff have put the implementation of standardized resuscitation protocols at the center of the subspecialty of emergency medicine.

Yet, although CPR protocols exemplify the benefits of the widespread implementation of procedural standards, they also indicate the mixed feelings professionals have toward the standardization of their work processes. An editorial in the prestigious medical journal, *Archives of Internal Medicine*, pondered the question whether a rule for the discontinuation of resuscitation is needed. Until now, no resuscitation protocol has indicated when resuscitative care should be terminated. The guidelines prescribe a minimum length but the decision to call it quits is the physician's prerogative. When discussing a proposed clinical decision rule for the cessation of resuscitative care, the editorial pointed to the clinical impossibility of predicting neurological deficits at the end of a resuscitative attempt. In addition, the editor warned: "Once a decision rule on futility of resuscitation is published, it quickly becomes a self-fulfilling prophecy. Therefore, asking whether the benefits of the decision rule outweigh the risks is important. There are economic considerations involved."[4] These economic considerations go beyond the cost of admitting a patient to an intensive care unit; they also relate to the cost for the profession as a whole. When noticing the self-fulfilling character of guidelines, the editor was afraid that once a rule had been formulated, the profession locked itself into it and lost clinical autonomy or its control over the decision to terminate resuscitative efforts. A new practice guideline might instead be used by insurance companies, for example, to determine the resuscitative care for which they are willing to pay.

Professions express a love-hate relationship toward standards in general, and clinical practice guidelines in particular. As explored in the introductory chapter, the history of modern medicine shows that the medical profession benefited greatly from the uniformity generated by recruitment, selection, and performance standards. Standards have been explicitly used to rid medicine of quacks, impostors, and alternative forms of healing and to put the human body under the jurisdiction of physicians, nurses, and other officially sanctioned medical groups. Currently, one of the main activities of the different colleges and academies in medicine consists of publishing hundreds of clinical practice guidelines to defend and explore new medical interventions and to diminish variation among its members. In this sense, clinical practice guidelines embody the extent of medicine's jurisdiction.

Yet, because clinical guidelines specify how to practice medicine, they also make professionals nervous. Such guidelines offer explicit instructions on which diagnostic or screening tests to order, when to provide medical or surgical services, how long patients should stay in a hospital, and other details of clinical practice. Telling members how to perform medicine is often construed as undermining clinical expertise and rendering the profession vulnerable to oversight, substitution, and interference. A survey of members of the American College of Physicians showed that while 70 percent of those surveyed thought that guidelines would improve the quality of care, 43 percent of the respondents believed that guidelines would increase health care costs, 68 percent believed that clinical practice guidelines would be used to discipline physicians, and 34 percent believed they would make medical practice less satisfying.[5]

In this chapter, we investigate the emerging politics of clinical practice guidelines on a professional level. We are interested in how the medical professions manage the potential of clinical practice guidelines to expand their jurisdiction while dealing with the danger that these same guidelines may weaken their professional and clinical autonomy. To simplify our analysis, we blur the differences between medical subdisciplines and employ a more generic notion of medicine. Following Andrew Abbott, Donald Light, and others, we look at how medical professions defend their jurisdictions in relationship with other social entities, such as the state, the insurance industry, allied groups, and liability lawyers. Our purpose is to work out how standardization helps shape a particular understanding of professional and clinical autonomy. *Professional autonomy* includes here the regulation of the profession as a whole by controlling entrance to the field, self-monitoring, developing a body of specialized knowledge, and running professional organizations. *Clinical autonomy* refers to the control the individual practitioner has over routine work activities and decisions, and the freedom to be innovative in the work process, for example, by prescribing drugs off-label.[6] Professional autonomy thus describes autonomy of an occupational group on an organizational level and marks the parameters for clinical autonomy. Traditionally, the litmus test for a profession's power is the autonomy its members have in their everyday work. Both kinds of autonomy are not pregiven characteristics but are negotiated and redefined through the interactions of many groups, resulting in the continuous redistribution of privileges and costs.

In the first part of this chapter, we explain how clinical practice guidelines reflect the relation of a profession to its work. The guidelines expand or confirm the scope of a profession's jurisdiction. In the second part, we discuss compliance of profession members to practice guidelines. We show that practitioners do not need to follow guidelines closely to advance professional goals. Incomplete compliance, however, creates vulnerability for professional and clinical autonomy because it opens a profession to external regulation. In the final part, we investigate what happens to professional and clinical autonomy when third parties hold the profession accountable to its own guidelines and try to enforce clinical practice guidelines for financial and legal purposes. We end this chapter with a discussion of how clinical practice guidelines helped transform the professional notion of autonomy into one of accountability.

CLINICAL PRACTICE GUIDELINES AND PROFESSIONAL JURISDICTION

What are the incentives for a profession to create clinical guidelines? According to profession scholar Eliot Freidson, standards help the profession protect a stock of knowledge from market competition, creating a "market shelter."[7] What distinguishes professions from other occupations is their control over the technical and formal content of their work. Andrew Abbott uses the term *jurisdiction*[8] and Donald Light *sovereignty*[9] to refer to the link between a profession and its work. Professions have relied on credentialing, registration, and licensing mechanisms to safeguard their jurisdiction against competitors and to avoid outside evaluation of their work.

Clinical guidelines are thus part of the formal body of technical knowledge over which a profession has unique jurisdiction. Among professions, "knowledge is the currency of competition."[10] Professional knowledge requires a balanced blend of abstraction (requiring special training) and specificity (concrete outcomes). Emerging professions competing with established professions have the most to gain from a more abstract system claiming a broad jurisdiction while established professions tend to refine and advance their knowledge more concretely. For both emerging and established professions, the work of generating professional knowledge is ongoing. In the same way that the new standards of the Dutch insurance physicians reflected changes in the disability laws, the body of medical knowledge needs to incorporate new scientific principles, technological improvements, and shifts in social context (scarcity of resources often leads to a tightening of decision criteria for expensive interventions).[11]

Established Professions

An important impetus for creating clinical practice guidelines for established professions is the clinical uncertainty, due to the vast amount of information. In the 1990s, an estimated 2 million medical articles were published yearly in more than 20,000 biomedical journals, more than 250,000 controlled trials of health care therapies had been conducted, and more than $50 billion was being spent annually on medical research;[12] between 1990 and 1995, for example, more than 14,000 articles in the field of hypertension were published on the topic of calcium-channel blockers alone. Another impetus is the partially corresponding practice variation that exists for particular medical interventions. Take, for example, the use of routine ultrasounds during low-risk pregnancies. Approximately 60 to 70 percent of pregnant women in the United States undergo ultrasound at various times during pregnancy without medical indications. Not only does the frequency of these ultrasounds vary (one to five ultrasounds over the course of a pregnancy), but questions exist about their sensitivity to detect fetal anomalies and risks to mother or fetus. Whether a pregnant woman will undergo an ultrasound, and how many, seems to be more dependent on a practitioner's personal preference or local customs than on sound scientific data, suggesting that some utilization might be inappropriate. The American College of Gynecologists and Obstetricians has recognized the potential for overuse of routine ultrasound and has issued an evidence-based guideline regarding the appropriate indications for routine ultrasounds during pregnancy.[13] The guideline is based on a literature review of randomized clinical trials performed over the past ten years. This evidence indicated that the sensitivity of a fetal anatomic survey to detect fetal anomalies varies widely, from 17 to 74 percent, and depends largely on the kind of clinical settings and the skill of the professionals performing the examination. In addition, the literature review did not conclusively settle whether fetuses with life-threatening anomalies have a better chance of survival after detection by routine ultrasound. The reviewers found that a reduction of perinatal morbidity and mortality and a lower rate of unnecessary interventions cannot be expected from routine ultrasound. In conclusion, "ultrasound should [only] be performed for specific indications in low-risk pregnancy."[14]

The routine ultrasound guideline is a professional tool because it originates from within a professional organization and is aimed at assisting members in their clinical decision making. Professional organizations refer to such guidelines as a "service" to their members: they sort the vast, specialized literature. Even when the evidence falls short of endorsing routine ultrasounds during low-risk pregnancies, the clinical practice guideline keeps the decision for ultrasounds firmly under the jurisdiction of obstetricians and gynecologists. It does not matter that obstetricians rarely manipulate the ultrasound probe themselves. The professional power that is confirmed here is the ability to evaluate a pregnant woman's medical condition and decide whether an ultrasound is indicated and interpret its results. The practice guideline positions obstetricians as the experts on prenatal diagnostic technologies, confirming their jurisdictional claim.

At the same time, the professional autonomy that is presented with practice guidelines instills a different kind of clinical autonomy from the one that dominated the past. Clinical practice guidelines try to reach the elusive fusion between scientific knowledge and clinical practice, attempting to turn the art of medicine into a science. Medicine has tried to become more scientific since the Enlightenment, but the intensity of this effort increased after the Second World War.[15] The construction of the atom bomb, the creation of radar, the discovery of penicillin, the revolution of the sulfa antibiotics, and cardiac surgery instilled an optimistic postwar enthusiasm that if one just devoted enough scientific brainpower and resources to a problem, a superior, rational solution was bound to be found. The result was a major infusion of money into academic medicine and specialized research institutes, the emergence of specialized research journals, a reorientation of medical education, and a full embrace of research values.[16]

Yet, observers kept pointing at the gap between the accumulation of medical knowledge and the application of this knowledge in the actual practice of most physicians. Sociological studies of the socialization of medical students showed that the ability to know the right thing to do was an almost intuitive sense of acting appropriately, a doctor's judgment generated over long years of doing "scut" work during intern-ships.[17] It accumulated with hands-on experience of a broad variety of patient bodies and learning the ropes of institutionalized practices. Clin-ical autonomy was the skill of rendering observed symptoms in indi-vidual patients meaningful to diagnosis and finding the therapeutic re-sponse most suited to this specific patient. Medical skills were acquired from role models at the bedside or in the autopsy room, and only secon-darily from textbooks. Clinical expertise always had a scientific ground-ing, but biomedical knowledge needed to be filtered through everyday, clinical experience.[18] Proponents of evidence-based medicine character-ize this now "traditional" medical paradigm by four assumptions:

1. Individual clinical experience provides the foundation for diagnosis, treatment, and prognosis. The measure of authority is proportional to the weight of individual experience.
2. Pathophysiology provides the foundation for clinical practice: diag-nostic and therapeutic reasoning relates symptoms and interventions to the underlying pathophysiological mechanisms that the physician infers to be taking place in the patient's body.
3. Traditional medical training and common sense are sufficient to en-able a physician to evaluate new tests and treatments.
4. Clinical guidelines are—at best—useful tools for novices, and—at worst—an unnecessary burden for the experienced physician. Clin-ical experience and expertise in a given subject area are a sufficient foundation to enable the physician to develop clinical practice guide-lines.[19]

The "new evidence-based medical paradigm" works under different assumptions:

1. When possible, clinicians use information derived from systematic, reproducible, and unbiased studies to increase their confidence in the true prognosis, efficacy of therapy, and usefulness of diagnostic tests. Clinical guidelines are necessary to bring this information to those places where clinical knowledge is applied: doctors' offices and clinical wards.
2. An understanding of pathophysiology is necessary but insufficient for the practice of clinical medicine. All pathophysiological infer-ences should be subordinated to the question of whether diagnos-

tic or therapeutic interventions have been proven to be effective in sound empirical studies.

3. An understanding of certain rules of evidence is necessary to evaluate and apply the medical literature effectively.[20]

In the current era, clinical expertise is the quality of an individual professional who practices methodologically and is not misled by unfound pathophysiologal inferences. Douglas Paauw asserts that many medical "myths" might make sense from a pathophysiological perspective but do not meet the evidence criteria. For example, students have been taught in major textbooks that giving narcotics to a patient with a possible acute abdomen syndrome may mask important signs and delay or even prevent an accurate diagnosis. Yet at least two controlled clinical trials found no difference in the accuracy of diagnosis between experimental and placebo groups.[21] The ability to palpate skillfully a patient's stomach or understand the pathophysiological course of action is losing its relative importance in comparison to the ability to search large information databases, assess the research reliability and validity of medical information, and discuss the cost-benefit probability of different treatment options with patients while keeping an eye on economic cost-effectiveness.[22]

The scientific model that clinical practice guidelines advance into medicine is overwhelmingly empiricist and grounded in epidemiological and statistical reasoning. What matters is to determine whether a (novel) intervention is more effective when given to a group of patients than a comparable (existing) intervention or a placebo. In other words, the aim is to determine whether the intervention has the diagnostic or therapeutic benefit it claims to have, and/or whether it works better than other interventions. How the intervention works, physiologically, or how, for example, contradictory results from different diagnostic interventions on similar patients should be understood is less relevant.

The ultimate criterion to establish scientific validity is a meta-analysis of randomized controlled clinical trials in which patients are randomly assigned to a treatment and a control group. The clinical trial was brought into general medical purview in 1946 when the British scientist Austin Bradford Hill designed the "first" randomly controlled trial to determine the effect of streptomycin on tuberculosis.[23] The clinical trial became institutionalized in the United States when the general public demanded governmental oversight because of the worldwide outbreak of birth defects due to the drug thalidomide.[24] The narrowly averted drug disaster in the United States led to stricter legal requirements for drug manufacturers to prove not only the safety but also the therapeutic efficacy of drugs (see Chapter 6). "By the late 1960s the double-blind methodology had become mandatory for FDA approval in the United States, and the procedure had become standard in most of the other Western industrial democracies as well by the late 1970s."[25] With the clinical trial, an experimental and probabilistic logic gained precedence over the pathophysiological postmortem and laboratory investigations of the past.

Thus, the professional agencies designing and refining clinical practice guidelines envision that these tools shorten the distance between accumulated medical knowledge and daily clinical decisions. The limits of the evidence-based physician's expertise are not the clinical uncertainty of the past but the limits of accumulated medical knowledge and a lack of familiarity with statistical methodologies. Sociologically speaking, the increasing societal pressures on the legitimacy of the medical profession's jurisdictional claims necessitated the introduction of statistically grounded "rules of diagnostic and/or therapeutic behavior."[26] Clinical practice guidelines give clinical autonomy a more deductive quality, based on general rules and statistical principles, instead of the more inductive and ultimately individually based skills emphasized in the past.

Emerging Professions

For less established professions, clinical practice guidelines are more often used to claim a special status and to solicit jurisdiction over a technical domain. The aspiring profession formulates clinical practice guidelines to stake out its special competence. A primary example of standardization with the explicit aim of advancing the professional goals of an emerging profession[27] is the Nursing Interventions Classification (NIC) developed at the University of Iowa.[28] This system of nursing tasks aims to depict and standardize the range of activities that nurses carry out in their daily routines. The third edition of this volume classifies a list of 486 interventions, each comprised of a label, a definition, a set of activities, and a short list of background readings.[29]

Each intervention thus forms its own clinical practice guideline. The system goes beyond a simple list of clinical guidelines, however. NIC aims to become the ultimate nursing standard: a standardized language offered as a list of standardized nursing interventions. The goal of the classification system is to render nurses' invisible, routine articulation work visible. A nursing researcher explained in an interview:

> A hospital administrator told me a couple of years ago: "If nursing could just tell us what they do?" You can't say "the nursing process" because everyone does nursing assessment, intervention. That is a model that everyone can apply. Physical therapy can say what they do: muscles and bones. Respiratory therapy can define their tasks. But nurses do all that. Nursing is so broad. The only thing that they know is that they can't work without us. NIC is extremely helpful because it provides a language to communicate what we do with a firm scientific base.

As a profession struggling under the tutelage of the well-established professional power of physicians, the Iowa researchers understand NIC as a necessary condition for nursing's survival. If the nursing profession does not define itself and claim a unique task packet, it runs the risk of disappearing from the health care map, to be replaced by poorly educated, part-time custodial workers or technicians.[30]

Like the ultrasound guideline, NIC is a professional tool, originating from within the profession, partly funded by professional organizations, and aimed at strengthening the professional position of nursing. But instead of requiring the randomized clinical trial as ultimate criterion of experimental science,[31] the methodology used by the NIC researchers is aimed at building consensus among profession members. While in evidence-based medicine "experts" determine the best way of performing health care, the NIC group built its methodology on a broad, explicitly democratic canvassing of the nursing profession. They surveyed compilations of discrete nursing activities and created a preliminary list, which distinguished between nursing interventions and activities. Expert surveys of nurses with master's degrees and focus groups narrowed the preliminary list of interventions. These interventions were further validated via surveys sent to specialist nursing organizations. Based on hierarchical cluster and similarity analyses, the different interventions were grouped and reviewed to assure clinical relevance and significance. The classification system is thus growing slowly through a widescale cooperative process, with nurses in field sites trying out categories and suggesting new ones and refinements in a series of regional and specialist meetings. Although the scientific process provides legitimacy, the aim of NIC is as much to unite nurses around a common task package as it is to provide a scientific bedrock for professional autonomy.

While concerned with preserving the clinical autonomy of individual nurses, the NIC researchers ultimately aim to carve out a distinct professional niche for nursing. This can be seen in the willingness of the researchers to expand the scope of their project to make even the most mundane tasks visible. Initially, the NIC group concentrated on direct care interventions, the tasks that benefit patients directly. The researchers deliberately supported an image of the classification of nursing as a clinical discipline. Several NIC team members noted the political nature of this decision in interviews. "Nurses think that laying hands on patients is nursing. We would not have had the attention of the nursing community if we had not begun there." Questions arose, however, in the course of the project about the distinction between direct care and indirect care (care that does not benefit a patient directly, such as filling out paperwork or maintaining supplies). Time spent on these tasks will be invisible if not included in NIC, and thus will be fiscally wasted. Over the course of the project, indirect interventions grew in importance and were included in the second edition of the NIC book.

The policy of the project managers has been to strive for completeness, revealing the full spectrum of nursing care. Yet, if the task that is brought under the scrutiny of terminological and procedural standardization is too obvious and mundane, then some nurses who are testing the system find it insulting. To tell a veteran nurse to shake down a thermometer after taking a temperature puts him or her into a childlike position. Some experienced nurses, encountering interventions they felt were too obvious, have called them an NSS, or "No Shit, Sherlock," intervention. To spell out even mundane tasks in minute detail calls into question the clinical expertise and autonomy of true professionals.

These grumblings of experienced clinical nurses have been secondary to the professional aim of rendering invisible nursing tasks visible, and defining the special expertise needed to do nursing tasks professionally. More than an intervention-by-intervention decision guide for nurses in their daily practices, NIC needs to be evaluated in its entirety.

The whole standardized system claims a set of tasks that are typical for nurses and it is this whole that forms the basis for the aspiring profession's jurisdiction and autonomy. The process of standardization by itself provides some level of legitimacy to the professional aspirations because it helps unite the diverse nursing profession behind a common set of nursing interventions.

Clinical practice guidelines thus endorse a profession's jurisdiction with a scientific and empirical base. In the contemporary health care climate, well-established, powerful professions rely on clinical practice guidelines validated by clinical trials to take stock of the available knowledge, reduce uncertainty and practice variation, and assist in decision making. Powerful professions are primarily concerned with optimizing and maintaining what they have, while occasionally also claiming new areas of jurisdiction. Less powerful and established professions primarily formulate practice guidelines to—in the case of nurses, inductively—stake out a claim of technical expertise and unite members. Their primary objective is to articulate a domain of expertise and appropriate new jurisdictions. The reliance on what is currently considered the "best" evidence, findings validated with randomized clinical trials, often remains out of reach for emerging medical professionals and medical practices at the health care periphery. Randomized clinical trials are labor intensive and expensive to run, they are tailored to particular patient populations (often not those regularly encountered in primary care, such as children and elderly patients), and do not apply easily to all clinical situations (how, for example, does one design a clinical trial for "cultural competency?").[32] One respondent in a study of alternative medicine noted that "it takes a lot of gold to meet the gold standard of the clinical trial."[33] Yet, for both emerging and established professional groups the process of standardization forms an attractive strategy to rally members and claim expertise. The corpus of procedural standards, including clinical practice guidelines, maps the area over which health care providers maintain professional sovereignty. The success of a profession to claim a tally of interventions with standards and clinical practice guidelines depends largely on the instruments' scientific backing. Issues of concern are the research and clinical validity of data, the process of guideline development, and the motives of the developers. To address these concerns, a new methodological literature is emerging that can steer professional committees through the abundance of medical research to come up with the best guidelines possible. Even if guidelines help confirm the scope of a profession's jurisdiction, how do these guidelines impact the daily practice of clinicians? Is the mere formulation of the scientifically best way to perform health care sufficient to change medical behavior? Next, we examine how clinical practice guidelines relate to clinical autonomy.

PROFESSIONAL "COMPLIANCE" WITH CLINICAL PRACTICE GUIDELINES

Clinical practice guidelines capture a profession's consensus on its area of expertise and suggest the preferred way to perform an intervention. They also fit in with cognitive theory: "they are intended to change behavior by providing definitive information on best practices from authoritative sources to well-trained, interested, logical practitioners."[34] One might therefore expect that the members of a profession would apply the guidelines consistently and overwhelmingly in their practice. This is not the case. Freidson noted that "standards accomplish an economic function by providing a market shelter for professionals *and at the same time leave the actual determination of the way work is done to them.*"[35] When clinical guidelines originate within professions, they might strengthen the professional infrastructure by providing authoritative model sequences of how particular interventions should be performed. But—and this is the most important characteristic of *professional* standards—individual clinical autonomy takes precedence over the normative and prescriptive aspect of the guidelines. As the complaints of the experienced clinical nurses to NIC showed, not all health care providers are willing to submit to the proposed order of clinical practice guidelines, especially if the WIIFM (what's in it for me?)[36] principle remains unarticulated.

Indeed, if we evaluate how clinical guidelines render actual behavior uniform in the way intended by their designers, these instruments have a diminishing rate of return. The general suspicion is that "guidelines may do little to change practice behavior."[37] Although inconclusive at best and weak when evaluated with EBM criteria,[38] most of the available research confirms this hypothesis. First, there seems to be little awareness of guidelines. A survey of 100 New Zealand general practitioners after the release of a guideline on the management of hypertension showed that only 40 percent had read the guideline.[39] Researchers in Seattle surveyed 300 pediatricians about their knowledge and impression of four well-publicized pediatric practice guidelines.[40] The awareness of the guidelines varied from only 15 to 66 percent, and the pediatricians dismissed the guidelines as too "cookbook," time-consuming, and cumbersome. Self-reported change due to the guidelines varied from 19 to 36 percent.

Second, even if known, clinical practice guidelines rarely change the behavior of professionals. A British study evaluating a clinical guideline for tonsillectomy for children found that before the standard was implemented 73 percent of the cases already conformed to the criteria of the guidelines, while 15 percent did not, and in 12 percent of the cases it was impossible to judge. After the guidelines were introduced, the statistics were virtually unchanged (73, 14, and 13 percent, respectively).[41] A Dutch case-review study of ten different practice guidelines found that clinicians followed the guidelines in 61 percent of the cases. For controversial decisions and "vague" guidelines, the average dropped to 35 percent, while guidelines demanding a change in practice routines were followed in 44 percent of the decisions.[42] A U.S. study checking a pneumonia practice guideline found no statistically significant effects of the guideline on patient outcomes, care following hospital discharge, and patient satisfaction scores.[43] The ability of an asthma guideline to change care providers' behavior was also found to be limited in the U.S. military when simply distributed.[44] Even if behavioral changes occur, they tend to peter out quite quickly, suggesting a "fatigue effect."[45] The overall compliance rate of clinical practice guidelines has been estimated at just more than 50 percent,[46] referred to in the literature as a "modest effect." Updates of the medical variance atlases show that after implementation of universal and even local standardized guidelines, the variance continues.[47] "The availability of evidence-based technology assessment is not enough to improve practice, reduce variation, and achieve better outcomes."[48] Two surgeons conclude, "The most certain statement concerning such guidelines is that physicians do not use them."[49]

Faced with the lack of behavioral changes, practitioners publish "guidelines for clinical guidelines,"[50] which set standards for the generation and formulation of guidelines. Also, they attempt to list the key traits for successful standard implementation and devote editorials to marketing techniques and the clinical learning process. The increased focus on guideline implementation includes education strategies, working with medical "opinion leaders," offering retrospective or concurring feedback, computerized clinical decision support, and one-on-one education of providers by commercial representatives or hospital pharmacists (the latter is referred to as "academic detailing" and is usually limited to drug prescription behavior), economic incentives for clinicians, and even offering patients money for following guidelines.[51]

When professions engage in guideline formulation, they bring authority to the guideline but even then their members look at guidelines more as options than as true standards. The profession itself does not enforce adherence to guidelines or reward guideline-following behavior from its members. Compliance to guidelines depends upon the fit between the standards and the goals and demands upon the individual health care provider. To qualify as practice guidelines for a profession, standards need to retain flexibility in clinical decision making. Freidson explains:

> Thus, by the nature of the process by which they are formulated and agreed upon, the vast majority of all professionally produced standards permit a significant amount of variation in products, services, and personnel policies on the part of the concrete organizations and professionals who are supposed to be governed by them. It is true that a norm is officially adopted, but it is not very restrictive.[52]

Not only do guidelines poorly capture the contingencies of everyday professional work, but they often specify tasks that are usually not performed by physicians themselves but are farmed out to "allied" professions. "The internal subordination of routine work is a characteristic strategy of professions claiming more jurisdiction than they can effectively serve, American medicine being the best example."[53] It is not exceptional to find nurses and technicians more knowledgeable than physicians about the latter's official jurisdiction.[54]

In and of itself, such noncompliance need not be a problem in the era of evidence-based medicine—as long as the rationale for disagreeing can be justified on scientific grounds. If clinicians decide not to follow guidelines, it should be because this specific case does not match the evidence underlying the guideline. In addition, there might be reasons to deviate from the guideline that are not incorporated in the evidence. If refusing an ultrasound might undermine patient loyalty of an expectant mother who is worried about her pregnancy, for example, an obstetrician will likely prescribe one even if there is no medical indication for the intervention. The creators of the ultrasound guideline explicitly recognize and legitimate such pressures when they add the disclaimer that "variations of practice, taking into account the needs of the individual patient, resources, and limitations unique to the institution or type of practice, may warrant alternative treatment or procedures to the recommendations outlined in this document."[55] In an appropriation of evidence-based vocabulary that turns the aims of EBM on its head, several physicians in David Armstrong's study of prescription behavior of psychiatric drugs stated that they conducted their "personal clinical trials" to decide whether the new generation of drugs were effective.[56] Or more generally, in the words of the editor of the journal *Evidence-Based Medicine*, "External clinical evidence can inform, but can never replace, individual clinical expertise, and it is this expertise that decides whether the external evidence applies to the individual patient at all and, if so, how it should be integrated into a clinical decision."[57]

Yet it is highly questionable whether the widespread noncompliance with evidence-based guidelines is indeed due to evidence-based considerations. At the very least, in all those cases that clinicians were not even aware of the existence of guidelines, their noncompliance cannot have been a conscious act! A growing body of research suggests that clinical practice guidelines are not well known or do not overwhelmingly change practice behavior in the way intended by the designers of the guidelines, whether supplemented by additional implementation strategies or not. All in all, evidence-based guidelines seem to be one of the many impulses pushing professionals in a specific direction— and a not particularly successful one at that. The continuing existence of so many other reasons to not follow guidelines is underscored in a spoof by two Australian physicians published in the *British Medical Journal*.[58] In situations when the available evidence is insufficient to qualify as evidence-based medicine, the authors offered seven alternative grounds for decision making: eminence-based medicine (base decisions on seniority), vehemence-based medicine (substituting evidence for browbeating your colleagues), eloquence-based medicine, providence-based medicine (letting the Almighty decide, less prevalent among surgeons), diffidence-based medicine (do nothing from a sense of despair), nervousness-based medicine, and confidence-based medicine (this category was restricted to surgeons). They must have touched a raw nerve because the *BMJ* readers offered a long list of additional alternatives, including effervescence-based medicine (practiced by physicians who have too much "bubbly" at the Christmas party), opulence (or profit)-based medicine, annoyance-based medicine, propaganda-based medicine, and arrogance-based medicine. These insider jokes underscore that standardized tools compete with many other motivations in decision making.

As we explained in the previous chapter, clinical practice guidelines are not simple input-output systems but coordination devices. What makes a clinical guideline a professional tool is exactly that active collaboration and submission are required. The professional needs to evaluate a clinical situation and sift through the patient's self-reported symptoms to single out what professional problem may be at stake. This in itself is a complex task marred by ambiguity and uncertainty, in which each physician relies on an idiosyncratic array of medical knowledge.[59] Next, the professional needs to decide whether a standard applies, or to decide which standard applies ("The nice thing about standards is that there are so many from which to choose").[60] Then the professional usually has leeway in determining which steps to follow and what outcomes to record, how to interpret the treatment regime and add in patient characteristics that might indicate compliance or success. As we have seen, however, this leeway is often rather large and the guideline's impact relatively small. In such a situation, the guideline's coordinating activity is restricted to the most minimal level of linking individual professionals—by the mere presence of these guidelines—into a collective of evidence-based practitioners.

How, then, do clinical practice guidelines affect clinical autonomy? If we take as criterion for success that clinicians apply guidelines whenever they might be appropriate, then the guidelines' rate of return is limited: very few guidelines would pass this test. This observation may not be a problem for the professions: as long as clinical practice guidelines are mainly perceived as an authoritative and scientific decision *aid*, their success in staking out claims to professional autonomy might not be dependent on their actual usage by physicians.

Even if practice guidelines do not generate the uniform behavior hoped for by their designers, it would be premature to conclude that they do not have any effect. Self-reports or studies relying on patient chart reviews might not pick up on the more subtle changes in clinical practice. There is a wide variety of use-modes of procedural standards: from a very strict following of detailed steps that would characterize a pilot's running through checklists to the outright ignoring of a guideline's "advice" that forms the other extreme. In between we find the more active guidelines described in the previous chapter, and the guidelines that do not become an active part of a practice's infrastructure, yet linger in the minds of the professionals involved. Such guidelines are constantly and routinely reappropriated in light of the organizational demands of medical practice and the situational requirements of each new case. They are hard for the researcher to spot, since they become part of a physician's or practice's ongoing work routines. Overall, however, instead of a radical change in behavior, the aggregated effect of clinical practice guidelines seems to be a more nuanced, ongoing learning process of ignoring, partially adapting, and partially implementing guidelines in a variety of ways. As we show below, often the effect of a guideline manifests itself more on a conceptual level than in crude behavioral change; guidelines help redefine the politics of accountability and autonomy. As long as individual physicians select which guidelines to heed and to what degree, the overall impact on their clinical autonomy will be minimal. Yet, this deliberate "noncompliance" might be changing rapidly, as we explore in the next section.

CLINICAL PRACTICE GUIDELINES AND EXTERNAL REGULATION

Every clinical practice guideline originating within a profession becomes a claim for professional jurisdiction aimed not only at medical practitioners but also at a number of other audiences with whom the profession interacts. In order to advance the cause of professionalization, clinical practice guidelines need to be externally recognized as the profession's jurisdiction. NIC researchers, for example, hoped that their classification of nursing interventions would allow a determination of the costs of services provided by nurses and planning for resources needed in nursing practice settings. They therefore encouraged the inclusion of NIC in health care computing systems, nursing curriculum reform, and public health databases. In interviews, NIC researchers noted that although nurses fill in for physical therapists during weekends, the nursing department is not always reimbursed for this service. Sometimes the money flows back to the hospital at large or to the physical therapy department, or these treatments are simply not reimbursed:

> [Nursing activities] are not a part of the patient's bill and nursing does not get credit for those dollars. My goal is to get nursing credit for those dollars and to have nursing seen as a revenue-generating part of the hospital system. Nursing care has always been a part of the room charge, and the room charge might change if we do these things. Some interventions that therapists charge for and nurses do as well, I think nurses should charge for, and that may show up on the patient's bill.

According to the NIC researchers, NIC will allow hospital administrators to determine nursing costs and resource allocation and stop such apparent freeloading.

This path of professional development is treacherous because the line between adopting and enforcing is easily blurred. For instance, it is possible that NIC might be used against nursing professionalization in some computerization and surveillance scenarios. Imagine a hospital administrator who has implemented NIC and evaluates what nurses are doing. In an effort to curtail costs and adequately allocate resources, the administrator might prescribe nursing activities that are more cost-efficient. When asked about this issue, a principal investigator emphasized that nurses need to address those questions anyway.

> It may create some problems, but it forces nursing into the mainstream and forces nurses to be responsible, accountable, health care providers. Then, of course, you have to deal with the questions that physicians have had to deal with for a long time. And we ought to be able to deal with that and find a good new solution.

The stakes of professionalization are raised highest when standards invade the financial and legal realm of established professions. If insurers pay for standardized provisions, the profession as a whole could score big gains. Of course, the profession can also lose if insurers decide that other groups or interventions are more cost-effective.

Here we enter the most contentious area of clinical standard development, which is at the very same time the main reason why practice guidelines have been championed recently. "Many believe that the economic motive behind clinical guidelines is the principal reason for their popularity"[61] or "Why such a strong interest in practice guidelines? The primary driving force is money."[62] Indeed, clinical practice guidelines are strongly associated with cost control. One of the largest volumes of clinical practice guidelines, the *Guide to Clinical Preventive Services*, has been incorporated by many insurers, managed care organizations, and employers to define preventive services benefits.[63] The ultrasound guideline mentioned above promised yearly savings from $350 million to $1 billion if physicians cut down on nonmedically indicated routine ultrasounds. The tug of war between professions and other powers changes dramatically when third parties seize clinical practice guidelines to hold medicine accountable.

In this context, a profession's "noncompliance" to its own guidelines creates a problem for the external validation of its jurisdiction. When the gap between clinical practice guidelines and actual practice becomes too large, the profession becomes vulnerable to attacks on its jurisdiction. Third parties can contest the profession's sovereignty or they can seize the clinical practice guidelines and hold the profession accountable to its own guidelines. In medicine, the second scenario has the largest potential to undermine both professional and clinical autonomy. Attacks may come from a number of parties. The most carefully watched development is the practice of utilization review prevalent in the managed care context of U.S. medicine. But government agencies in Europe and Canada have also turned to clinical practice guidelines to regulate medicine. The recent white paper on the new National Health Service from the British Labour government, for example, rests upon the application and promotion of evidence-based medicine to obtain "clinical governance."[64] Yet in Europe, these modes of external regulation are still few and often shortlived. In the next section, we first discuss managed care in the United States, and then turn to a Canadian example.

United States

The surge of managed care has instituted cost-containment by controlling health providers as the organizing principle of U.S. health care. Physician organizations have expressed deep concern about managed care's insertion of a third party between the professional health care provider and the patient, second-guessing the professional and undermining the patient's trust in her or his health care provider's motives. Of particular worry is managed care's frequent reliance on third-party utilization review, "which typically is portrayed as undermining the medical profession by unduly standardizing medical practices or by creating excessive distractions and burdens for clinicians."[65] Utilization review organizations oversee physicians' use of health care services for more than 100 million people.[66] Instead of a simply retrospective fee-for-service system in which an insurer pays for the services deemed necessary by a health care provider, in utilization review a health care provider needs approval from the utilization reviewer before a procedure or service can be administered (prospective reimbursement).[67] Physicians are required to provide extensive documentation of diagnostic tests for every request in the hope that care provisions will be covered. The reviewer (usually a trained nurse) judges the medical necessity of the request and either denies or approves it. The treating provider and the patient have the right to appeal the noncertification. Board-certified clinical peers, actively working in the same profession and similar specialty as a provider, consider appeals.

The U.S. federal government initiated the first form of utilization review in 1972 as an attempt to monitor the ever-burgeoning Medicare and Medicaid programs. The practice then spread to the private health care sector.[68] Initially one or more physicians or nurses examined the medical record and judged the length of stay and appropriateness of requests using implicit criteria, but increasingly utilization review is guided by standardized guidelines. The Appropriateness Evaluation Protocol (AEP), the Standardized Medreview Instrument (SMI), and the Intensity-Severity-Discharge (ISD) criteria are examples of the standards used to evaluate the severity of a patient's illness with the level of service requested.[69] These instruments differ from each other in their organization and in the number and content of the criteria included. Reviewers are allowed to over-ride the instrument when they believe the assessment is inaccurate. Some of the utilization review standards are developed in-house while others are adapted from the guidelines developed by professional organizations and the government.

A survey of 109 utilization review firms showed that "review practices threatened autonomy most frequently through standardization."[70]

The researchers identified 14 percent of the surveyed firms that more than the others attempted to impose uniform national criteria. These "severe" firms were called "standardizing review organizations":

> Standardizing review organizations are most likely to act to transform prevailing clinical practice. Although they respond to the concerns of individual clinicians, they are not supportive of local practice norms, are associated with intrusive review processes, and allow their physician reviewers less discretion than do other review organizations. Interestingly, these are also the organizations in which the medical director and medical staff have the most pronounced influence over organizational policies.[71]

Standardizing utilization review firms are also more likely than the average firm to contact patients on a regular basis, as well as to warn them about inappropriate treatment that might threaten their health. Standardizing firms are thus the most aggressive at protecting the well-being of individual patients (against physician mistakes or oversights) and the most active at reshaping clinical practice. These firms also had the highest denial rates of claims submitted (14.1 percent versus an average of 6.7 percent) and make little or no adaptation to their review criteria based on clinicians' complaints. Although more than half of the firms use the information to profile individual physicians and hospitals for adverse outcomes, few report this information to professional regulatory bodies.

According to the critics of managed care, standardizing firms magnify what is endemic to utilization review in general. These third parties have shaped clinical and professional autonomy in at least four ways. First, *the utilization reviewers change the nature of practitioners' work.* They add to the administrative burden at the expense of direct patient-physician interaction. Physicians report that they spend more time on the phone, negotiating with utilization reviewers. Pocketsize booklets such as *A Physician's Guide to Utilization Review* provide physicians with lists of "Do's and Don'ts" of how to chart a patient's condition strategically and improve the chance of having a procedure approved.[72] The consequence is an increase in costly administrative time, often at the expense of direct patient care.

Second, *the utilization review firms challenge clinical autonomy directly when they decide whether an intervention is medically necessary, imposing changes in the content of medical work.* Although great variation remains between the proportion of hospitalization requests that are accepted,[73] the fact that permission is required from a third party means that clinicians are not in full control of their work. Utilization review firms determine whether, how, and how long a patient can be treated. In addition, the firms will contact the patient directly when they suspect that care was insufficient, again undermining professional autonomy. Ultimately, utilization review firms are also able to gather utilization profiles of individual practitioners and determine which physician or hospital is the most cost-effective. In theory, utilization review could be aimed at quality enhancement but in reality it seems to be used predominantly for cost control. Researchers found that Medicare carriers used guidelines to identify providers who provided overly sufficient care and to motivate them to lower costs and not to provide better quality care.[74] Utilization review removes Freidson's protective professional "market shelter" for exposure to internal and external competition.

Third, *utilization review indicates a shift in the status of the clinical practice guidelines.* With utilization review, the voluntary, flexible guidelines are more likely to become normative. Financial reimbursement adds accountability under the form of financial incentives or penalties to the structured physician-patient encounter.[75] The consequence is that clinical guidelines run the risk of becoming self-fulfilling prophecies. Physicians are hired, compensated, disciplined, and terminated by provider organizations based on their adherence to guidelines. "It must take a particularly scrupulous and principled physician to maintain what he/she believes are appropriate quality standards in the face of evidence that they are on the path to censure, economic credentialing, and exclusion from provider groups for implied resource overutilization."[76] Instead of guidelines, clinical practice guidelines increasingly attain the status of normative rules. For that reason some professional organizations now hesitate to write clinical practice guidelines.[77] The American College of Obstetricians and Gynecologists offers a strongly worded disclaimer at the end of its "criteria sets": "Use of criteria sets alone as utilization review criteria or to deny payment may represent an inappropriate use of these documents."[78]

Finally, *utilization review affects professional autonomy because the review agencies are willing to go beyond the profession to create guidelines.* The companies create their own guidelines, adopt them from government agencies, or alter professional guidelines, sometimes enforcing them over the objections of the medical profession. Utilization review organizations also instituted guidelines where professional organizations did not consider it necessary or possible to create guidelines. This undermines the knowledge base of the profession. An example of this can be found in an HMO Quality of Care Consortium funded study, where the researchers developed their own clinical practice guidelines for hysterectomy (the surgical removal of the uterus), the second most common surgical intervention in the United States (after caesarean-section). Hysterectomy rates are infamous for their geographic variation.[79] Yet, the American College of Obstetricians and Gynecologists has not created any prescriptive clinical practice guidelines, presumably because of the great uncertainty in the medical community about the indications for hysterectomy.[80] Using their own criteria generated from a panel of nine managed care physicians, the researchers funded by the RAND Corporation evaluated seven health care plans and decided that on average 16 percent of the hysterectomies were unnecessary.[81] Although in this case the guidelines were used to evaluate health care plans, the possibility also existed of evaluating physicians and practice collaborations (called practice profiling or benchmarking).[82]

Canada

In the United States, the increased prevalence of clinical practice guidelines was stimulated by private, market-driven parties inserting themselves between patient and clinician. The same effect can be obtained from government intervention as a Canadian case study shows. In the Canadian province of Ontario, the Ontario Medical Association (OMA) championed clinical practice guidelines to regain the government's and general public's trust after a contentious physicians' strike in 1985.[83] In order to avoid the introduction of blunt utilization control instruments, the OMA intended to develop voluntarily, flexible guidelines, incorporating "sensible" (from the perspective of the professional) economic evaluation, but driven by the need for quality of care rather than fiscal constraint.

Such initiatives quickly broke the physicians' ranks and undermined professional autonomy. To the surprise of radiologists and cardiologists, the province physicians' organization argued against the introduction of new, expensive radiology and cardiology techniques. The OMA also collaborated with the government on the formulation of cholesterol guidelines more conservative than those promulgated by the Canadian Consensus Conference on Cholesterol and apparently embarrassed the medical profession by publishing an atlas of regional variances in medical utilization. Although the cholesterol and other guidelines were mailed to every physician, few practitioners seemed to comply with them because of their close association with "government medicine." Instead of strengthening the medical profession, the lack of compliance with the clinical guidelines undermined professional solidarity. OMA specialty sections accused the larger organization of undermining their expertise. Conservative physicians considered the OMA's collaboration with the government on guidelines a threat to clinical autonomy. The OMA accused the government of not providing a financial incentive for guideline compliance. When an economic recession hit Canada in 1992, the government in turn instituted across-the-board reductions of physicians' income, resulting in physicians overbilling their patients. "Surely the OMA's worst fear, that blunt utilization control mechanisms would detract from professional control over the content of care, was realized when physicians altered their clinical decision-making to compete with each other for personal income."[84]

The important consequence of the Canadian guideline movement was a loss of clinical autonomy and professional solidarity on a macro level. The government gradually increased its control over medical service utilization, bypassing the OMA altogether when evaluating the introduction of new technologies and stepping up its requirements for prior approval for insured services.[85]

The managed care industry and government agencies are not concerned with preserving professional or clinical autonomy but with holding medical practitioners *financially accountable*. Sociologist Donald Light has referred to this movement as "the revolt of payers."[86] Fed up with the exploding costs in an unchecked fee-for-service system, increasing distrust of physicians' values and competence, assumed quality of health care, overspecialization, excesses and inconsistencies in care, and fragmentation of services, the payers in the health care system have tried to monitor and control physicians' practices.[87] Autonomy requires trust that professionals will practice on behalf of patients, but with this trust largely eroded, accountability became the watchword. Yet holding someone accountable requires some basis for judgment. Rather than merely checking someone's credentials, or just acting upon patients' complaints, clinical practice guidelines offer third parties the missing bar to pry open the black box of clinical judgment. Guidelines provide reformers with a tangential set of tasks for which outcomes can be measured, providers can be compared, and a cost-benefit analysis can be undertaken.

An important advantage of guidelines is that they are scientifically validated. Gary Belkin analyzed managed care's reliance on scientifically derived standardized measures as a manifestation of the *"technocratic wish,* an appeal to objective measures to resolve contentious issues and/or clothe their resolution as scientifically logical and natural."[88] He adds, "Managed care may represent a transition from epistemological to instrumental standardization, from using standard measures as tools for more accurate knowledge about disease and treatment, to relying on such scores, protocols, and algorithms for their instrumental convenience in managing the needs of large numbers of people."[89] In our view, Belkin underestimates how "epidemiological" standards are necessarily politically active and how not only managed care organizations but all interested parties—notably the medical professions— rely on the epistemological, instrumental, and authoritative potential of guidelines. But he is correct in pointing out managed care's active role in stimulating epidemiologically based guidelines to wrestle authority away from physicians.

Therefore, these government and private utilization reviewers build their reforms of medical practice around clinical practice guidelines and intend to hold practitioners accountable by offering incentives as well as disincentives. While boosting clinical practice guidelines and refining standards of practice, these external parties do professional work for the professions. They develop practice guidelines and fund the research that underlies them, boosting the evidence-based nature of medical work. While third parties dovetail on the authority professional committees bestow on guidelines, they also bypass the profession and formulate guidelines that are unacceptable to professional members. In 1989, Freidson already described how the emergence of standards and (standard-based) formal review procedures could reduce the individual physician's autonomy in determining the content of her or his work. Yet Freidson stressed how these standards and procedures were made and executed by *other physicians*—not by outsiders.[90] In this analysis, the medical profession would maintain its *overall* professional autonomy position by reinforcing a stratification *within* the profession: "New modes of evaluating and exercising control over the work of [rank-and-file] physicians are created by reinforcing and formalizing the positions of medical administrators or supervisors and of medical researchers."[91] During the next decade, however, the fact that the control over the work of the rank-and-file physician remained internal to the medical profession would become more and more contested.

Based on loud, indignant protests from clinicians in medical editorials and the popular media,[92] the financial threats of third parties seem to have been quite successful in changing medical practice and enforcing clinical interaction backed up with scientific evidence. The threat of cuts in income or reimbursements, or the restrictions on physicians' choices, created an incentive for health care providers to pay attention to clinical practice guidelines and actually follow them. But while the rhetoric might be heated, it is still unclear whether these pressures led to consistent and widespread change in clinical behavior. For example, economic incentives remain the least studied of the different guideline implementation interventions and the few studies do not reveal consistent statistically significant behavioral changes.[93] The strongest impact of third-party pressures might be indirect: third parties might help the implementation of guidelines by offering reimbursement for the services and time commitments required in the guidelines, that is, by creating a guideline-friendly climate.[94]

CLINICAL PRACTICE GUIDELINES AND THE LAW

Increasingly, clinical practice guidelines have played a role in U.S. tort law to establish liability, deter future harmful conduct, compensate injured victims, and challenge the determination of what benefits are covered under a health plan. Here, evidence-based medicine moves into the legal realm, possibly morphing guidelines into tools of legal accountability. In American courts, disputes are resolved in an adversarial system that allows each party to submit evidence and bring forth experts most favorable to its legal claims, and to cross-examine, discredit, and rebut the expert witnesses of opposing parties, leading to the "battle of the experts."[95] Judges are supposed to admit evidence that is relevant, probative, and not prejudicial to parties.[96] When the opposing parties dispute the facts, the responsibility of sorting through the evidence and determining what facts to believe is left to a jury of laypeople or to a judge acting as a lay fact finder. "To establish medical liability, an injured patient must show that the physician failed to exercise the appropriate standard of care owed to that patient. . . . The medical profession sets its own standard of care based on what is customary and usual practice, as established through physician testimony and medical treatises."[97]

Some health care observers have noted the transparency provided by evidence-based medicine in the adversarial legal system with increasing concern: "EBM is seen by some as packing a one-two punch: erosion of autonomy going into a treatment situation accompanied by greater risk of liability after the fact."[98] Indeed, the different interpretation of "evidence" in the legal and medical realm points to the risk of equating evidence-based medicine with the legal standard of care.

> Regardless of which party in the dispute introduced the guideline, however, the litigation always casts the same issues into especially bold relief: the conflict between the impersonal objectivity of a guideline and the personalized expertise of the physician, or the conflict between the guideline's focus on general decision procedures and the legal (and medical) profession's focus on the particular facts of the case under consideration.[99]

The director of the Agency for Healthcare Research and Quality, John Eisenberg, lists six differences in the legal and medical views on evidence.[100] First, in court, evidence refers to what caused harm to an individual or might have been denied the opportunity for benefit from actions not taken. In other words, evidence in courts is deterministic, used to assess and assign responsibility. In clinical practice informed by evidence-based medicine, evidence is probabilistic and based on large population studies. Second, physicians use evidence to determine a future course of action, while in court evidence is interpreted retrospectively, to determine the causation of a harmful event. Third, in health care a new treatment might take years to diffuse with clinical practice guidelines recommending practices that might differ from the practice of most physicians, while in the legal realm, legislative action or precedent-setting decisions by judges might more drastically change legal practice. Fourth, evidence in medicine and science is determined by a peer-review process, while in the legal realm lawyers decide what evidence to submit and judges decide what evidence the jury will hear. Consequently, in law juries determine the validity and reliability of evidence presented to them while in the health care field experts themselves determine what constitutes valid evidence. Finally, in both areas the rules of evidence remain in flux and make it difficult to calculate the legal ramifications of services based on guidelines alone. Some observers have therefore called for a federal certification of clinical practice guidelines.[101]

At stake is thus how courts treat the practice guidelines when determining the professional community standard in a medical area. No conclusive pattern has emerged in the way courts regard clinical practice guidelines, but it is likely that guidelines may gain importance if widely adopted and followed by the medical community. The attraction for courts is that practice guidelines are developed systematically, are scientifically validated, are issued by an authoritative organization, and often express the consensus of a medical subdiscipline on a minimal standard of care. If the courts find the guideline definitive as standard of care, the guideline becomes the yardstick against which a physician's practice is judged. Clinical practice guidelines can be used to immunize physicians from malpractice liability, but failure to comply with guidelines can expose them to liability, rendering guidelines "two-way streets."[102] Physicians might, for example, be able to dismiss lawsuits when they can document adherence to clinical practice guidelines, but the burden of persuasion might also shift from the plaintiff to the physician who did not adhere to existing practice guidelines. Because of the great variability in development and use of practice guidelines, the American Medical Association opposes the direct adoption of clinical practice guidelines as a legal standard and urges that they should only be entered as evidence.[103]

Although clinical guidelines can be used by plaintiffs and defendant physicians, there is evidence that practice guidelines are used more for inculpatory purposes (by plaintiffs) than they are used for exculpatory purposes (by defendant physicians). Researchers surveyed two malpractice insurance companies, 600 randomly selected malpractice attorneys, and the legal literature to ascertain the frequency and nature of the use of clinical practice guidelines in malpractice litigation.[104] Guidelines were successfully used in twenty-eight cases. Twenty-two cases used inculpatory guidelines compared to six cases with exculpatory guidelines. Guidelines from the American College of Obstetrics and Gynecology, the American Psychiatric Association, and the American Academy of Pediatrics were used most frequently for inculpatory intent. In the survey, malpractice attorneys also reported that once a lawsuit is initiated, practice guidelines are more likely to be used for inculpatory (54 percent) than for exculpatory (23 percent) purposes, and 30.9 percent reported that clinical guidelines influenced their decision to bring at least one lawsuit during the previous year.[105]

The use of clinical practice guidelines in court to inculpate physicians might undermine the guidelines even before they are established. Physicians might not want to develop or adopt guidelines out of fear of liability consequences. Proponents of clinical practice guidelines have successfully lobbied for state laws allowing only exculpatory use of the guidelines (rendering them "one-way" streets). In this situation, the guidelines serve more as regulator. Yet, Arnold Rosoff warns that "allowing such one-sided use of evidence in a court of law raises disturbing questions of fairness and of validity under the U.S. Constitution's Fifth and Fourteenth Amendments' due process and equal protection mandates, and under state constitutional principles as well."[106] The use of guidelines in court cases also makes unfamilarity with guidelines problematic: "How embarassing and damaging to a physician and/or surgeon on a hospital staff who has never read the hospital's practice guidelines to find that practices that have served in good stead for 30 years are no longer considered the standard of care and may be used against that particular individual in a malpractice case."[107]

The court's attitude is still marred with ambiguity regarding whether clinical practice guidelines constitute definitive standards of care. Most observers anticipate that "courts will treat clinical practice guidelines as one piece of evidence in establishing the standard of care, rather than as the primary determinant of the appropriate standard of care."[108] The adoption of clinical practice guidelines in legal doctrine again changes the status of the guidelines. Instead of offering voluntary assistance in clinical decision making to improve patient care, physicians might feel pressured to adhere strictly to the guidelines although adherence might both reduce and increase liability. Some malpractice insurers are mandating compliance with guidelines as a condition of coverage or are threatening surcharges or cancellation if a claim results from not following guidelines.[109] As a consequence, articles in health administration journals encourage the close adherence to clinical practice guidelines to avoid or lower liability.[110]

TOOLS OF ACCOUNTABILITY?

Clinical practice guidelines simultaneously constitute a profession's heart and an Achilles' heel. The establishment, protection, and expansion of a profession's jurisdiction might change clinical and professional autonomy and open a profession up to accountability to a third party. Professional organizations deliberately develop criteria to improve quality of care, reduce practice variance among practitioners, and preserve the profession's control over the content of medical care. When insurers, governments, and courts are in a position to enforce clinical practice guidelines by linking them to physicians' incomes, however, accountability might prevail over autonomy. The accountability that is aimed for depends on the transparency of health care interventions: the best evidence renders interventions observable and by implication subject to attempts at control. Using financial incentives and penalties third parties attempt to tell health care professionals when and how to perform or not to perform certain interventions. This particular kind of accountability goes to the jugular of professional autonomy; it attempts to regulate the decisions health care providers take in their daily work.

The most common forms of regulating professions is to make decisions about the allocation of resources to patient care and management on a national, regional, or institutional level, and to limit the clientele of professionals by formulating criteria that qualify for reimbursement or, more generally, by instituting rationing procedures.[111] While all forms of accountability have in common that health care professionals are held accountable to third parties for the value of health care, the newer form of accountability attempts to manage the entire clinical process by making it transparent. "In countries with a national health care system administrators and policymakers can use guidelines to assign resources to areas where they are needed the most. In countries with a private-based health care system, plan administrators and insurers can use clinical practice guidelines to make decisions about what services to authorize (i.e. reimburse) for patients with given conditions."[112]

The consequence of using clinical practice guidelines as professional tools is that both the nature of the guidelines and the professional's autonomy are redefined. First, the nature of the guidelines changes. Clinical practice guidelines always need to strike a balance between precise prescription and allowance for leeway. Guidelines prescribe one way of doing medicine over others, while at the same time leaving a certain margin of discretion to make its application feasible. Even in the strictest guideline, the practitioner still has to decide whether the guideline applies in this situation.

When professional organizations formulate clinical practice guidelines, their authority frames the prescriptive character of the instruments. The evidence-based methodology, consensus of experts in the field, and the aura of the professional organization further enhance this. Physicians were more likely to follow guidelines formulated by the American College of Physicians than those created by the insurer Blue Cross-Blue Shield (even though both institutions have collaborated on guidelines).[113] But the profession does not want to impose clinical guidelines on its members. A professional organization does not offer any rewards for the professional whose practice best exemplifies guideline following, neither does a penalty exist for repeated deviation from guidelines. Instead of highlighting the prescriptive nature of guidelines, professions emphasize the educational and decision support function of clinical practice guidelines. Physicians learn about guidelines from reading journals, speaking with colleagues, logging on to web sites, and going to conferences. They juggle the requirements of the guidelines against the contingencies of patient care. From a profession's point of view, clinical practice guidelines do not determine but guide their behavior.

Outsiders—government agencies, private insurers, and courts—attempt to strike a different balance. Third parties are not in a position to prescribe medical behavior; professionals largely determine the content of their work. Outsiders, though, can try to hold the profession accountable to its own guidelines. Dovetailing on the professional authority already invested in the guidelines and the valued scientific process underlying the guidelines, these outside parties will try to enforce the prescriptive nature of the guidelines and erode the leeway granted to professionals to appropriate them to their own situations. The key mechanism for such conversion is financial accountability. The outsiders build incentives to tie guideline-following behavior to the care provider's wallet. Clinical practice guidelines become the standard to which medical behavior gets measured in utilization reviews and figures in the determination of the legal standard of care. Outsiders aim to turn professional guidelines that merely guide behavior into standards that prescribe it.

With the introduction of clinical practice guidelines, the meaning of professional and clinical autonomy has also shifted over time. The profession's introduction of clinical practice guidelines provides a scientific, evidence-based rationality for professional autonomy. When third parties seize clinical practice guidelines to regulate medicine, clinical autonomy gives way to accountability. What is at stake is who decides how medical work should be done. Are the people trained to do the work or those who pay in charge? The 1950s and 1960s are often considered the "golden age of doctoring" in the United States and elsewhere in the Western world because of the large autonomy physicians had over the entire medical realm.[114] Bolstered by surgical and pharmaceutical breakthroughs, physicians medicalized and practiced with little resistance, knowing that they would be reimbursed by insurers and the government in a fee-for-service system. When the excesses of this system became known and trust eroded, third parties preoccupied with the excessive costs of health care tried to get a handle on the content of health care work.

Some critics view the external reinforcement of clinical practice guidelines as a further indication of the medical profession's deprofessionalization, corporatization, or even proletarization.[115] But using terms like *deprofessionalization* and *proletarization* supports a static, profession-centered view of the world. These concepts presume that autonomy is a quality that only decreases or increases, instead of a characteristic that is historically situated. In addition, because of the evaluative connotation of the terms, gaining autonomy is considered a positive evolution. Light notes that autonomy is actually a form of professionally immunized accountability: "Rather than being the irreducible core of professionalism, autonomy is a second-best substitute for accountability, long used because one could not look inside the black box of clinical judgment and therefore had to grant the profession autonomy and trust that members would use it to maximize patient's well-being."[116]

Viewed in this perspective, clinical practice guidelines are a missing link for a redistribution of accountability. They are the new weaponry in the tug of war over professional jurisdiction. The question is whether their effects resemble an ongoing skirmish or the touted last big battle. For now, it seems too easy to circumvent third-party control as physicians have done when the government instituted diagnostic-related groups (DRGs). The use of DRGs involves reimbursing hospitals a flat sum for each Medicaid patient they care for, regardless of individual diagnosis or length of stay, but based on the broad category in which the diagnosis falls. If physicians want to maintain their income, they can join forces and engage in "appropriate referrals" (also known as cost shifting to someone else's budget), market segmentation, market expansion, and service substitution. "All are easier and often more profitable than trying to become more efficient, particularly when the work is complex, contingent, and uncertain."[117] Other studies have shown repeatedly that "physicians react to fee freezes by increasing volume."[118] Similar appropriations of the clinical guidelines likely abound in utilization review or other forms of regulation. Indeed, one of the important observations is that even with strong financial incentives clinical practice guidelines do not seem to change providers' behavior in a consistent manner.

While clinical practice guidelines might have opened the black box of clinical judgment for third parties, those parties have not been able to break the monopoly of professionalism. The key problem that remains is changing the networks in which the health practices are embedded, a lesson that both the professions and third parties keep learning and that goes back to the heyday of scientific management and Elton Mayo's Hawthorne experiments of motivation. Implementation experts decided that the success of clinical practice guidelines in changing behavior depends on the quality of the guidelines, characteristics of the health care professional, characteristics of the practice setting, incentives, regulation, and patient factors.[119] In such a list of variables, even strong financial incentives might not generate much change. EBM advocates rely for implementation strategies on the technique they know best: the randomized clinical trial, to test different ways of effecting change. Where the drug trial is aimed at providing a treatment for disease, clinicians are perceived to have impediments to behavioral change that require an intervention. But it "seems highly unlikely that a simple behavioral intervention can displace the complex cognitions that anchor a clinical repertoire in the everyday experience" of clinicians.[120]

Indeed, we wonder—along with other observers—whether the days of clinical practice guidelines as a preferred policy tool to improve health care delivery and control costs might not be numbered.[121] After spending millions of dollars on nineteen guidelines between 1992 and 1996 with little measurable results of changed physician behavior, the U.S. Agency for Health Care Policy and Research retreated from guideline development, profiling itself more as a clearinghouse and sponsor of guidelines.[122] HMOs have also come to the conclusion that "clinical guidelines alone may not be sufficient tools of quality assurance for children with chronic or complex conditions"[123] and the promised cost-savings of guidelines have been largely unfulfilled.[124]

While clinical practice guidelines with more or less voluntary participation might not necessarily be the best tools to shift practice patterns and limit costs in the long term, they seem to have a persistently subtle effect on professions. The process of standardizing generates and confirms an explicit sense of professional identity. The creation of clinical practice guidelines involves a process of delegation to experts or unity through wide-scale surveying of professional members and, most important, a scientific stock-taking of what the profession is all about. In assessing the strengths and weaknesses of available evidence and tallying the areas of expertise, a professional group makes its own jurisdiction internally and externally explicit, offering a rallying point for research, education, reimbursement, and so on. The process of standardizing itself is thus an important indicator of professional assertion, and, as we have seen, established and emerging professions have different priorities and follow different procedures to generate standards. At the same time, the final product of the standardization effort crystallizes a perspective of the boundaries of professional expertise. Such statements often reconceptualize the position of the health care provider, the subjectivity of the patient, and presumes a secondary role to third parties. In the chapter that follows, we explore how insurance physicians reconceptualize the objectivity of their work and what they and their patients are about.

4   Guidelines, Professionals, and the Production of Objectivity in Insurance Medicine

IN THE previous chapter, we focused on different ways in which evidence-based guidelines present themselves as double-edged swords for the professionals and professions that encounter or generate them. The same activities that may enhance the scientific image of a profession might reduce clinical autonomy; the instruments that make the profession's decision-making processes more transparent also may make that process more vulnerable to meddling by outsiders. In this chapter, we zoom in on one specific case to investigate these issues further: the introduction of guidelines in insurance medicine in the Netherlands. We investigate how insurance physicians defined and perceived these guidelines, how they felt these instruments affected their work, and how their professional position was implicated. In this appraisal, we bring two new points of attention into the analysis. First of all, we look at the role the notion of objectivity played in these developments. We argue, put briefly, that a redefinition of objectivity played a key role in the active alignment, by the insurance physicians' profession, of the processes of guideline development and professionalization. Second, we focus on the way the patient was defined in these guidelines. The redefinition of objectivity simultaneously implied a specific conceptualization of the position of the client in the insurance physician's work. Different standards, we argue, not only affect professionals and professions differently: they may embed different notions of objectivity (and therefore what constitutes sound and scientific medicine), and they can define the role and position of patients in significantly varying ways.

At first glance, objectivity seems to be one of the central goals of evidence-based guideline development that necessarily incorporates

the tension between enhancing and threatening a profession's autonomy. Clinical practice guidelines aim at increasing the base of objective
evidence underlying health care work, at increasing the transparency
of medical practice, and at reducing unnecessary practice variations.
As such, they may strengthen a profession's status by increasing, for
example, its perceived scientific character. They do this, however, by
enhancing transparency (and thereby facilitating external influences),
reducing the subjective aspects of health care work, and limiting the
maneuvering room of individual professionals and clients. Enhancing
the objectivity of work practices through the introduction of procedural standards, then, would seem to be a hazardous strategy from the
perspective of the profession involved.

For the position of the patient, such a notion of objectivity would be
similarly problematic. In the insurance physician setting, patients are
often referred to as "clients," emphasizing the importance of an equal
relationship (as little as possible based on unilateral dependence). The
insurance physician should serve the client as much as is possible within
the institutional and legal frameworks of her or his job. On the one hand,
then, the increased transparency and improved possibility of external
control that a more objective claim evaluation could offer might be seen
as a step forward toward a more equal positioning of patient and professional. On the other hand, however, the emphasis on following standard
procedures, based on scientific evidence, could also leave precious little
room for patients to influence the course of their own care trajectories.
Moreover, an emphasis on objective evidence might direct the physician's attention even more to laboratory tests and other objective measures of the patient's condition, and belittle even more the importance
of the patient's own story and experiences.[1]

Recent sociological and historical studies of science have shown how
objectivity is a term that means different things in different times or situations. In their study, Daston and Galison demonstrate how the modern
notion of objectivity mixes several historically and conceptually distinc-
tive components. Notions such as empirical reliability, procedural correctness, emotional detachment, being true to nature, and being without
perspective are all intermingled in our current usages, which are epistemological as much as moral.[2] Similarly, other authors have shown how
the notion of objectivity varies between different scientific fields[3] and
how the specific notion of objectivity that emerges in a certain era or

area should be seen as related to the social and political circumstances that were prominent in that era or domain.[4]

In addition, the objectivity of a fact or activity is no longer seen as a quality of that individual fact or act. Rather, the objectivity of a fact is a quality of the historically and locally specific network to which this fact is attached.[5] X rays, for example, only became objective through the standardization of X-ray equipment and photographic material, through the training of technicians, through the construction of boundaries between normal and pathological, and through the stabilization of links between X-ray images and other diagnostic technologies.[6] Objectivity, then, is an effect of a network that can vary across times and spaces, not a universal characteristic inherent to an entity or process. This implies that objectivity might be a capacity that is open to negotiation and redefinition—and that, therefore, might not necessarily lead to the reduction of discretionary space for individual professionals and clients outlined above.

In this chapter, we draw upon this theoretical background to elucidate how the tensions between professionalization and guidelines in this field were mediated by a redefinition of what it meant to judge objectively a social insurance claim and a redefinition of what patient faced the insurance physician. We interviewed insurance physicians, coordinating physicians, and general managers from four different administrative bodies.[7] Coordinating physicians supervise the work of insurance physicians, and are responsible for keeping up the professional quality of their work (through introducing national guidelines in their offices, for example). The general managers are the directors of regional offices of the administrative bodies, which employ the physicians and are responsible for the actual allocation of disability benefits. In addition, we did a text analysis of the four procedural standards we studied (the first standards introduced in the field by the National Institute for Social Insurance [Lisv], which formally functions as the contractor of the administrative bodies).

In the first section, we introduce the specific practice and guidelines under study. Subsequently, the general reception of these guidelines by practitioners and general managers is discussed. These paragraphs sketch the background to the third section, in which we discuss the redefinition of objectivity that figured prominently in this development, and the repositioning of the patient.

THE PRACTICE AND THE GUIDELINES

As already discussed in the second chapter, insurance physicians have a crucial role as gatekeepers in the Dutch social security system. For those social security arrangements that deal with disability, such as the Disability Benefits Act, the medical evaluation of an insurance physician is a central step. In evaluating a claim, the insurance physician investigates whether and how much the current medical condition of the client hinders this client from doing work. The insurance physician consults a so-called labor expert about the specific capacities required for a certain job, the financial implications of a reduction in capacities, and so forth. Both insurance physicians and labor experts are employed by administrative bodies that are commissioned by the recently created National Institute for Social Insurance to carry out the allocation of benefits (the institute is ultimately responsible for the cost and quality of the services performed by the administrative bodies). In drawing up the contracts with the administrative bodies, the institute consults both unions and employers' organizations. Like the administrative bodies themselves, these are organized per sector: one administrative body deals with civil servants, another with workers in the construction industry, and so forth. The premiums for the Disability Benefits Act are paid by employers and managed by the institute.

Because of the relatively large numbers of individuals receiving a disability benefit in the Netherlands, the functioning of the Disability Benefits Act has come under intense public scrutiny. In 1993, in a parliamentary inquiry into the execution of the Disability Benefits Acts, the labor and employers' organizations were accused of using the Disability Benefits Act to get rid of redundant employees without rendering them formally unemployed (unemployment benefits are much lower). Insurance physicians were accused of going along with these practices, of being too easy, and of failing to uphold their gatekeeper function. They were an easy target: both from within and outside the medical profession, insurance medicine is seen as ranking low on the status ladder of the medical profession.[8] Insurance physicians have no curative tasks; they can only evaluate claims, assist in the prevention of disability, and help clients return to the workplace.

The parliamentary inquiry symbolized the attempts of the government and parliament to get a grip on the social security system and to reestablish public control. It stimulated the reorganization of financial responsibilities in the field and the formation of new institutions for the administration and management of the social insurances (National Institute for Social Insurance)[9] and their public control (Social Security Supervisory Board).[10] The inquiry led to the introduction of many new acts and generated continuous debate about the possibility of privatizing parts of the public insurance system. In relation to this, the culture of social insurance in the Netherlands underwent a major transformation. While in earlier times the social insurance system was geared primarily toward paying the benefits in time—because it was supposed that disability was a qualification for life—now the reintegration of the sick and disabled became a primary aim. In line with this transformation, a legalistic, administrative, bureaucratic social security system had to develop into a system in which much more than administrative work has to be done in order to stimulate actively the reintegration of sick or disabled employees in the labor process. These developments are still ongoing. In the meantime, the numbers of people receiving a benefit have not diminished substantially since the inquiry: in a total population of less than 15 million in the Netherlands, the number of people receiving disability benefits is over 900,000. Politicians follow these developments with impatience and continuously propose changes in the prevailing acts and organizational setup. The Dutch social insurance field remains in turmoil, and most parties involved still feel insecure about the way it will develop further.

This also was the case when we did our research in 1997. The physicians we interviewed were insecure about how their work would develop in the near future. The reorganization of social security, for instance, went together with calls from politicians that only the really disabled should have a legal claim on benefits. This notion resulted in an enforcement of the distinction between real medical problems and all the other, more vague reasons people could not function anymore (such as psychosocial complaints). Within this line of reasoning, insurance physicians, no matter how badly they might have functioned in the recent past, were still seen as the central gatekeepers to social insurance. However, the reorganization of social security and the novel emphasis on reintegration also led some politicians and administrators to argue that physicians need not be all that central to the social security system and that other specialists (such as labor experts) could have a larger role to play.

As an explicit strategy to enhance the quality and transparency of the work of insurance physicians, the National Institute for Social Insurance, founded in early 1997, continued the guideline program that had been set up two years earlier by its institutional predecessor. In the 1997 description of the central goal of its guideline policy, the social pressures figure prominently. The guidelines have to

> enhance the quality of the claim evaluation by specifying the professional activities of labour experts and insurance physicians. Through standardizing the activities of labour experts and insurance physicians, it should become easier for clients and third parties to gain insight in the claim evaluation process. This has to result in a more open and controllable claim evaluation practice, which will ultimately enhance the quality of the service.[11]

Quality, in this definition, implies meeting legitimate expectations and needs of both legislator and client; it implies meeting both professional and legal criteria. The following aspects of quality are distinguished: timeliness, completeness, correctness, and proper treatment (of the client as person).

Uniformity of processes and criteria is mentioned as well, because this would also enhance the insight and the equity of the claim evaluation (NLAP standard). Strictly speaking, the dissemination and integration of evidence into the delivery of care, a core aim of the evidence-based movement, is not the central aim of the guidelines studied here. The guidelines deal with topics for which no randomized controlled trials are available, and there is no formal procedure for incorporating other types of evidence into the construction of the guidelines. Yet the guidelines do attempt to bring the best possible professional and legal insights into the practices of the insurance physicians. Likewise, the scientific mind-set required from the insurance physician, and the attempt to enhance uniformity and quality of professional services, is central to the evidence-based movement. What should be rendered uniform are the methods and evaluation criteria that should result in a "timely, complete, correct and properly treated" claim evaluation.

At the time of our study, some ten procedural standards were at work within the claim evaluation practice, and more standards were in development. The institute attempts to closely involve the insurance physicians and the labor expert in the development of standards. No formal development programs (as the consensus meetings common in curative medicine) exist, however; the guidelines are developed in small working groups, installed by the National Institute and consisting of interested insurance physicians from the different administrative bodies. The four standards studied here were the standards that were introduced first.

The four guidelines that we focused on are as follows:
• *The guideline medical disability criterion (MDC)*
In the 1993 Dutch Disability Benefits Act, the criterion for disability was defined as "unfit for labour as a directly and objectively determinable medical consequence of a disease or infirmity." The MDC guideline attempts to translate this legal requirement into a framework that can guide the practitioner in the evaluation of actual claims, and aims to break the automatism with which physicians often reason from the presence of illness to the presence of disability. Briefly put, the practitioner is asked to investigate the presence and mutual consistency of *disturbances* ("of physical or mental structure or function"), *limitations* (in daily functioning), and *handicaps* (in social roles, especially the role of laborer). Only when handicaps directly follow from limitations that, in their turn, directly follow from disturbances can there be labor disability. This guideline is presented almost as an essay, outlining the philosophy underlying claim evaluation. The legal requirements and the political discussions leading up to the exact phrasing are recounted in detail, and several pages of text are used to explain and illustrate how the terminology of disturbances, limitations, and handicaps should be understood and used.
• *The guideline "no lasting available possibilities" (NLAP)*
This guideline delineates a number of conditions in which the insurance physician can judge a client fully unfit for labor without having to investigate precisely the mental and physical capabilities of the client (and to create a so-called task capacity profile [*belastbaarheidsprofiel*] to determine the client's capacity to work). Such conditions are, among others: admittance to a (mental) hospital, being bedridden, or "incapacity to function personally or socially." This guideline is brief and less philosophical, and is accompanied by a brief "version for practical use": a thick A4 sheet, on which the guideline is summarized in text and (on the other side) in a flowchart (see Figure 4.1).

Figure 4.1. Flowchart from NLAP guideline

Method of the standard with regards to prognosis

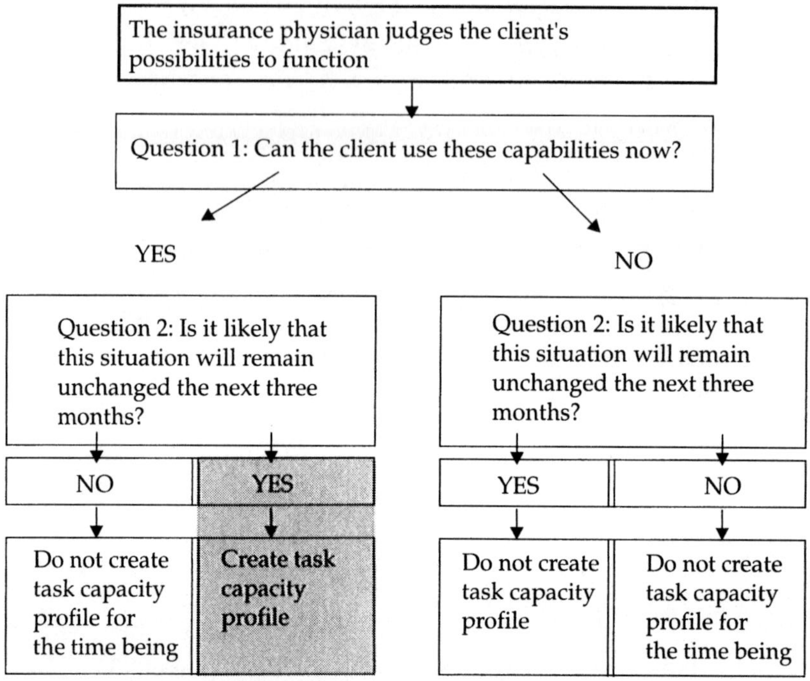

Source: NLAP work document.

• *The guideline "cooperation labor expert and insurance physician" (CLIP)*

This guideline outlines the procedure of a labor disability claim evaluation that is not one of the exceptional cases delineated by the previous guideline. It lays out the mutual responsibilities of labor expert and insurance physician, and designates moments when consultation is called for. This guideline consists of several pages of text, explicating the responsibilities and consultation moments in relatively abstract terms.

• *The guideline "increased labor disability 'due to identical cause'" (ILD)*

This brief guideline aims to determine whether or not a change in labor disability status can be seen as due to the original cause or not. Whether or not this is the case is important for complicated legal and financial reasons: if the condition of a partially disabled employee deteriorates, the employer is *not* financially responsible if the increased disability is due to the "same" cause. This guideline has been distributed in the form of a two-page letter with two brief appendixes to insurance physicians and administrative bodies.

These four briefly described guidelines are intertwined in complex ways. In curative medicine, guidelines usually focus on specific diagnostic or therapeutic situations. In an ideal case, such guidelines would cover the whole realm of medicine without overlap, so that in every clinical case there would be just one guideline that is operative. The guidelines we just described, however, *all* overlap. The first two apply in all labor disability claim cases—MDC outlining the general approach that needs to be taken, and NLAP summing up a list of special cases in which the task capacity profile does not have to be made. The last two guidelines also both fall within the overall MDC framework. CLIP specifies the normal consultation procedure between insurance physician and labor expert in claim evaluations, whereas ILD focuses on one specific category of claims.

"TEN CLAIMS PER DAY": THE OVERALL RECEPTION OF THE GUIDELINES

The guidelines we studied were all introduced in the years 1995–97. The precise status of the National Institute for Social Insurance guidelines was not always clear to all parties. Whether they were guidelines that suggested optimal paths of actions, or whether they held a particular legal status and could be enforced was not clear. The institute itself spoke of "constraining policy instructions," a description that in its ambiguity (and in its lack of clarity about how the constraints would be enforced) did not help much to resolve this confusion. Overall, however, the insurance physicians and general managers we interviewed were positive about the guidelines, pointing at the uniformity and equity that they would help to bring.

How can we explain this positive reception? The double bind between professionalization and guidelines—enhancing its scientific base, while potentially also reducing its maneuvering space—exists in this field just as much as elsewhere. Managers and professionals did not necessarily agree on *why* guidelines were such a good idea. The following quotation from a general manager illustrates the view that many health care professionals find rather chilling:

> Guidelines outline quite precisely when one can ask for a return visit from someone, and for what reasons. That used to be much less prescribed, and an insurance physician could shape the evaluation and rehabilitation process whichever way he wanted. I think that standardization is good. It makes the [work] more professional, I think. Not everyone will agree. . . . a few people who are attached to the rehabilitation and the soft side in their job will probably have trouble with this. They will not see this as a positive development. Yet I think it is an improvement; the clearer, the better. Those that do not like this, and that goes for everyone, should reconsider whether they want to stay in this job. (PM)

In this view, guidelines result in tight and standardized working patterns, a development subsequently equated with professionalism. This is not a view that many physicians would hold. Why, then, did so few physicians interviewed speak of the dangers of guidelines, or the threat of standardization?

One explanation is that the introduction of the guidelines was seen in the light of the increasing need for public legitimization of the profession of insurance physicians. The physicians and managers we interviewed both felt that the public criticism of the implementation of the Disability Benefits Act had made clear that something had to happen:

> The standard was implemented in a time that the general atmosphere was that the Disability Benefits Act had run out of control. The atmosphere was that . . . we needed a grip to get a hold on things. The general feeling was that something needed to happen, otherwise things would go really wrong. I think that that helped to have these protocols be made and accepted. (PE)

Instruments such as guidelines could help prevent carelessness and arbitrariness in the claim evaluations. Managers stated clearly that they believed in uniformity: "If you see a physician in Maastricht or in Dordrecht, that shouldn't make a difference" (NM). Or, as another manager phrased it: "I think you owe it to society to ensure that you perform your tasks with a certain level of quality" (AM). Likewise, the physicians stated that the guidelines provided clarity and a framework, a "grip," to hold on to (PE).

As argued in the previous chapter, relatively weak professionals such as insurance physicians might indeed embrace guidelines as a potential means toward higher professional status.[12] Through generating guidelines, the profession could show outsiders that they take their task seriously, and that they can be trusted to handle claims responsibly and justly. One insurance physician indicated that the MDC guideline had helped insurance physicians stand more firmly in their interactions with employers, employees, and managers:

> For a long time . . . there was a culture of not being difficult, just signing that [the claim for disability] was medically justified [whenever that was asked from you]. Then a disability benefit could be given. . . . [With the guidelines] you challenge that culture a little, you have to give reasons: that is why someone is and that is why someone is not unfit for labor. So I think that you limit your freedom, but you increase clarity, and you reduce the possibility for doctors to just go along with a deal to "prevent being difficult." Fifteen years ago, for example, people were declared unfit all too easily. Just signing the forms, going along, was the norm. With the current standard, that would have been impossible. (PE)

The MDC guideline, according to this physician, gave doctors an additional argument to claim their own professional jurisdiction, and to withstand pressure from others—such as employers, the physician's general manager, and clients. In this way, the guideline both strengthens the insurance physicians' profession and yields a more strict enforcement of the law: because physicians take their own, independent role more seriously, less clients will be entitled to a disability benefit.

A second reason for the physicians' lack of negative reactions to the institute's guidelines was that they more often than not matched the working patterns as they had emerged after the parliamentary inquiry:

> [The standard is] a reflection of what had been our practice for a while already. So in that sense I have not modified my way of working. But everything did get more explicit, it did become clearer: you have to clarify the consequences [for the ability to work], and make explicit how these consequences result from illness. (PE)

This match was due to the fact that the guidelines were made in close cooperation with the insurance physicians in the field:

> The [NLAP] standard was developed by a collaborating group and there has been much feedback from the field. In our staff meetings, for example, we have often discussed this standard when we would receive new drafts. [The outcomes of these discussions were] brought back into the working group, and so forth. We've actively participated in making that standard. So it is rather logical that we find it usable. (DC)

Third, physicians indicated that they were not afraid of the guidelines because these tools did not take away the need for their professional skills. Evaluating disability claims, the physicians interviewed stressed, was a complicated, highly delicate process, in which issues were rarely clear-cut:

> Say someone has lower back pain. . . . The complaints are worse because there are tensions in his home situation. It is evident that he'll not be at ease there. It isn't always black and white; sometimes there are subtle aspects that come into the picture. [To make a decision between a client] who "does not want to work" or one who "is not able to." . . . It isn't that black and white. (RE)

Many complaints or afflictions defied easy measurements or clear-cut decision criteria:

> Consider the chronic fatigue syndrome. That's all very individual. You have to listen to what the client tells you: is that a consistent story? And you have to ask information from the family doctor, and then again you have to make a judgment: is that or isn't that consistent? That remains difficult, whatever you do, you can't simplify that. (AC)

The institute's guidelines, it was felt, acknowledged this complexity of the decision process. The guidelines were seen to leave a space for interpretation and judgment that could only be filled by the specific knowledge and experience of an insurance physician. They did not do away with the need to think:

> They don't make it lighter, like "I no longer need to think because I can just apply the standard." That's not how it works. Whether you apply a standard or figure it all out for yourself, you have to balance carefully what you do, and that hasn't changed. (IE)

The guidelines, in fact, left the physician quite a range of possibilities:

> [The standards] aim at a standardized approach and at uniform results, but they remain dependent on the professional know-how and judgment of the insurance physician. The MDC guideline, for example, states that you have to ask the patient how he spends his day. You do that, as you should, and you note "he spends the whole day on the couch." Subsequently I do not get the impression that this patient is actually depressed. Nor does he seem anxious, [and I do not find anything else wrong with him either]. You could say: he spends his whole day on the couch, so he has no lasting available possibilities, because he doesn't leave the couch. You could focus on that, let him lie on his couch and be fully unfit for

labor, while you could equally focus on everything you do not find, and everything that is still OK and then you say: he is still fit to work. I could draw both conclusions on the basis of this same protocol. (NE)

In the following quotation, the coordinating physician expresses the expectation that the existence of this discretionary space safeguards the clinical autonomy of insurance physicians while not limiting the guidelines' effectiveness in defending their professional jurisdiction vis-à-vis relevant outsiders:

> Standards will always leave some room for your own autonomy. They leave enough space, I think. . . . I hope, for example, that at court, the judge will be more easily convinced when we point at the standard . . . and that the judge then says, OK, I agree with that. That would enhance our autonomy, I think. (RC)

In line with these remarks, some physicians objected to the term *standards*, which was sometimes used to denote the institute's tools:

> They shouldn't become straitjackets . . . I prefer the term *guideline* over *standard* . . . *Guideline* sounds like this is the overall direction, which leaves more room for my own interpretation. *Standard* sounds so definite, like "the only way and the only truth." (IE)

An important reason for the insurance physicians' positive stance toward the guidelines, then, was that they felt that these tools left a space for professional judgment. In fact, one physician argued that the threat to the profession's autonomy did not so much come from guidelines but from bad management:

> You hear emergency calls from doctors who feel their office no longer allows them to work in what they feel is the professionally right way. You have general managers with a vision, and you have [incompetent managers] who just seem to find pleasure harassing the doctor. Always make a full task capacity profile, no reinvestigations, ten disability claims per day. (NE)

In general, however, insurance physicians did not appear to feel overly controlled or regimented by their coordinating physicians or general managers. There was no sense of a "fixed, structured supervision" (PE). The increased attention to their functioning had not led to an increasingly tight line of command or surveillance within the administrative bodies. Nor were guidelines used as a means to steer the work of insurance physicians: "It's not giving me any trouble," one physician put it (DE).

Because the guidelines left room for professional jurisdiction, and because guidelines were not used by coordinating physicians or general managers to increase their control over insurance physicians' work tasks, they felt that more was gained than lost in submitting themselves to the standard (see Chapter 2). As much as setting the norm for the professional action of insurance physicians, their professional insights set the norm for the application of guidelines: "If I would apply these standards literally then I would violate my own judgment about how to evaluate a situation" (IE).

CHANGING THE DEFINITION OF OBJECTIVITY AND PATIENTS

When it comes to the status of a profession, we have argued, guidelines are a double-edged sword. They can bring an aura of science and quality, yet they can simultaneously result in external control and loss of clinical autonomy. Especially in an already relatively weak profession, the introduction of guidelines by a national agency that is *not* an association of professionals might seem to be a rather controversial enterprise. Yet we did not encounter much resistance to the guidelines in our research. One reason why this was the case might have been the specific context in which Dutch insurance physicians work. Much more than their colleagues in curative medicine, it could be argued, they are used to working in a strongly bureaucratic and judicial environment, the current transformations toward a focus on reintegration notwithstanding. Novel rules delineating their work, then, might not be as foreign and threatening to them as they would be for curative physicians. The arguments in the previous section, however, indicate that this is not a suitable explanation. For these physicians, the image of a practice meticulously prestructured through fine-grained protocols by managers and other third parties figured just as much as a horror-scenario as for their curative colleagues. The guidelines, rather, were felt to be a necessary response to the increased public pressure on their profession. They could act as a resource in legitimating their work—for the public, as well as for individual negotiations with employers, employees, and other parties involved in a particular case. The guidelines were felt to be acceptable, moreover, because they mostly matched the working routines as they had been recently established, and because they left a space for interpretation and judgment.

For the insurance physicians, then, the guidelines materialized the idea that their work was not just routine and predictable in the sense that almost everybody should be classified as legitimately disabled. In the context of the specific transformation of the Dutch social security system—from the administration of benefits payments to an emphasis on reintegration of the sick and disabled into the workforce—the introduction of guidelines explicitly acknowledged that physicians had something to decide. They were not just puppets on a string, acting according to the consensus of employers and employees, but they really had a complicated job to do: to distinguish between legitimate and illegitimate claims and to determine the degree of disability. In fact, the guidelines expressed the difficulties of the job as they had experienced them since the parliamentary inquiry.

In this section, we would like to take a further, in-depth look at how the insurance physicians were able to manage the tensions inherent in the attempt to professionalize through the development of guidelines. Both the National Institute and politicians who worried about the problems in the claim evaluation process hoped that the introduction of guidelines would make that process more objective: more transparent, more controllable, and more scientific. How, in this politically charged environment, in which the personal interests of the insurance physicians could not be expected to carry much weight, did guidelines emerge that were felt to actually strengthen their position? In a move that would make many a philosopher of science jealous, the authors and users of the guidelines *redefined what objectivity meant* in such a way that the potential tensions between enhanced objectivity and professional autonomy evaporated. In the same movement, these authors redefined what it meant to be a patient, or client, in the insurance medicine setting. They underscored both the need of a clinical autonomous professional and the centrality of the patient's story in the process of claim evaluation. There are two components to this impressive act of practical philosophy, and we discuss them in turn.

For the first component, let us return to the guideline "medical disability criterion," the overarching guideline that sets the framework for the other ones. This guideline recounts how the legislator has changed the medical disability criterion from "unfit for labour as a consequence of a disease or infirmity" into "unfit for labour as a directly and objectively determinable medical consequence of a disease or infirmity."

Accompanying this change, the minister for social affairs and employment announced that it should be seen as a signal that the concepts *disease* and *unfit for labor* should not be interpreted too loosely. The claim evaluations had to become more stringent, although this should not be taken to imply the exclusion of, for example, psychosomatic complaints that are difficult to prove unequivocally. Given this legal base, the MDC guideline attempts to create starting points for the medical claim evaluation by "interpreting the medical disability criterion."[13] This implies that the insurance physician is asked to investigate the presence and mutual consistency of disturbances, limitations, and handicaps. The criterion is met only if the disturbances directly lead to limitations "in meeting the demands of the work tasks in question," and if the disturbances, limitations, and handicaps are "objectively medically determinable." This latter phrase, it is explicated further, means: observable, in a controllable and reproducible manner, by the insurance physician through means "generally accepted in health care." Through this definition, it becomes possible to "objectively medically determine" social and psychological problems, syndromes such as chronic fatigue syndrome, and complaints from, for example, hernias that are hard to measure. In other words, the phrase "objectively medically determine" is interpreted in such a way that the experiences and perspective of the client take a central position in the claim evaluation. An overly biomedical focus on diagnosis is not what the insurance physician should be after, the guideline argues. To the contrary: being unfit for labor is often a complex matter with multiple causes and reinforcing and alleviating factors, including matters as diverse as "labour conflicts," long travel times, and "dangerous hobbies."

In this interpretation, to "objectively determine" a complaint is not taken to imply that only that which can be quantitatively measured, or unambiguously observed, is valid. Rather than opting for this frequently encountered interpretation of objectivity, the authors of this guideline are at pains to *redefine objective determination to mean the controllable and reproducible interpretation and weighing of a wide range of medical, psychological, and social considerations.* Doing so, the guideline does not force the physician to use one type of test, or to pose one series of questions. Rather, the guideline implies that a broad array of tests, questions, and methods can be relevant in the determination of medical disability. Biomedical tests, stories, the consistency between the patient's story and the physical examination, information from the general practitioner—the insurance physician can select from all these elements to create and substantiate his or her claim evaluation. There is no hierarchy between these elements: quantitative laboratory results, for example, are not privileged over qualitative interpretations about the family history. The guideline posits them as equal, and privileges or excludes none.

The guideline thus creates a space for the insurance physician to balance this array of arguments and considerations against each other in evaluating a medical disability claim. The MDC guideline reads the Disability Benefits Act in a particular way: through a specific definition of objective determination, a broad range of considerations remains valid, the patient's perspective remains central, and the insurance physician's maneuvering space is enlarged rather than constrained. Through this redefinition of objectivity, the aims of guideline development and professionalization have become perfectly aligned rather than potentially at odds. Whereas guidelines usually delineate what procedure to follow in a specific situation, and thus inevitably impinge on the physician's clinical autonomy, this guideline actually succeeds in creating and safeguarding latitude. Contrary to Freidson's analysis,[14] we see here guidelines that help to safeguard the jurisdiction of the insurance physicians' profession *while at the same time creating more rather than less leverage for the individual rank-and-file professional.*

Yet the MDC guideline cannot be merely seen as a strategic move in a battle for professional jurisdiction: it is simultaneously a move in an ideological debate about how claims should be evaluated and what the role of the client should be in the claim evaluation process. In these guidelines, the client is positioned as an active, responsible actor, whose self-interpretation and experience should figure as core input for the insurance physician. The client, in other words, should not be seen as an object whose status is to be assessed through external means, but as a person who is most directly implicated in the whole situation, and whose perspective should therefore be central. This position is not primarily a political statement about the importance of the client-as-person. First and foremost, it is a position that recognizes the client as the central agent within any attempt to prevent or limit a prolonged trajectory of labor disability.[15] In this ideology, treating the client as a responsible subject is the most proper and efficient way to stimulate him or her to (partially) return to the labor process.[16] Importantly, the guideline puts the client central while retaining an independent plat-form from which to judge the patient's accounts and activities. The pa-tient is put central, in other words, yet the insurance physician does not operate solely as a patient's advocate—which would be unacceptable for a gatekeeper who is under fire for being too lenient.[17]

The redefinition of objectivity, then, serves multiple goals, which re-turn in the other guidelines. In the guideline "increased labour disabil-ity 'due to identical cause' " (ILD), for example, the physician needs to determine medically and objectively whether a change in labor disabil-ity status is due to the cause that originally resulted in disability or not. If a person is partially disabled due to a heart condition, for example, and becomes fully incapacitated due to a major heart attack, it is clear that the "original cause" also caused the increase in labor disability. If the person would have developed a stroke, however, or in the case of many psychological problems, this determination is not so easy. In line with the philosophical framework of the MDC guideline, this guideline interprets the objective determination of the original cause as follows: a "reasonable case needs to be made" that the current limitations follow "predominantly" from the original cause. When uncertainty remains, the guideline continues, the client should be given "the benefit of the doubt." Here again, objective action by the physician implies carefully weighing a wide range of diverging considerations in full awareness that clear-cut causality is the exception rather than the norm.

The only guideline that does specifically prescribe how to act in a specific circumstance is the guideline "no lasting available possibili-ties" (NLAP). This guideline is the only one that actually contains a list of explicit decision-criteria, and that is represented as a flow-chart (see Figure 4.1). It outlines the situations in which it is not necessary to investigate precisely the mental and physical capabilities of the client (to make a task capacity profile). In such a case the client is immedi-ately deemed to have "no lasting available possibilities," and is thus eligible for a 100 percent disability benefit. Here, the objective determi-nation of disability is given shape through a circumscribed list of pre-defined situations: if the patient is bedridden, for example, or resides permanently in a (mental) hospital, the criteria for NLAP is automat-ically met. In this guideline, then, objective action is interpreted in a way that at least partially conflicts with the overall MDC philosophy: here, objective determination implies the mechanic following of pre-explicated rules.[18]

Not surprisingly, then, it is exactly at this point that many interviewed physicians raised concerns. A fixed list of conditions can only lead to unjust situations, they argued. There are many situations that do not figure in the explicit list in which it was nevertheless "obvious" (to the experienced insurance physician) that there are "no lasting available possibilities." In such situations, the guideline would force the physician to complete the formal task capacity profile—which is much work, and can be a heavy burden for the patient:

> I had somebody with a brain tumor and according to the [guidelines] his task capacity had to be estimated to match him to labor tasks he could still perform. That man could no longer talk properly and did not have a clue what type of headache he had: his wife had to come with him. He had a switch in his hand, through which he could add drops of chemo[therapy] into his blood or something. Can you imagine? According to the [guidelines] the insurance physician should have completed a full task capacity profile. That man is now dead. (NM)

In such cases, the physicians complained, the guidelines hampered the quality of their work. Here, objective determination was given a too mechanistic and rigid meaning, limiting their clinical autonomy and harming the client. When they encountered such a client, the physicians stated, they let their judgment prevail. They either ignored the guideline, or rewrote the patient's story so that one of the criteria was met after all. As one physician put it: "Often you see that a professional comes to a judgment, and then writes it either into or out off the standard" (NE).

Except for one part of one guideline, then, the authors of the guidelines consistently interpreted objective determination as the client-centered balancing of a wide range of considerations and information. This is the first ingenious way through which the aim to make the claim evaluation more objective was aligned with the professionals' desire for self-determination. The second way, which is equally ingenious, returns us to the meaning of such terms as *observable, controllable, reproducible,* and *transparency.* Whereas the redefinition illustrated above was a clear feat of the guidelines' authors—it could be traced in the text of the guidelines—this second way of redefining objectivity was also a matter of the way insurance physicians interpreted the guidelines in their work.

For a large part, the guidelines attempt to enhance the objectivity of the work of insurance physicians through requiring more explicit and more extensive reporting. In this way, the claim evaluation process would become more transparent to both clients and other third parties. Through the explication of the decision process, the physician's task performance would become more open and, in that way, more controllable. Although the guidelines themselves also went into much detail about the shape that the decision process should take, many interviewees mainly emphasized that the guidelines changed their reporting practices. They used to be "much briefer" (RE):

> The standard ensures that you substantiate your opinion. You need arguments . . . Before, a report about back complaints might just say: "the complaints are real, limited heavy carrying"—that was the whole report. The standard forces you . . . to objectify and collect arguments why you feel that a person with back complaints should only be allowed to lift five kilos. It should be convincing and logical. (PE)

In fact, several interviewees stressed that the increased attention to reporting was the main or even the sole effect of the guidelines. The guidelines, according to these physicians, result in more extensive reports, which in its turn makes their judgment verifiable. The *content* of their judgment, however, "that what he does" has not changed; "you only write it down differently" (HC; RE).

As above, this way of enhancing objectivity can likewise be typified by the absence of constraints on the physician's decision-making process. A focus on more explicit and extensive reporting, in other words, is quite different than restructuring the decision process itself, for example, or outlawing subjectivity through strictly limiting the types of considerations that might be allowed. All these alternative routes *could* have been taken under the flag of increasing objectivity—yet the routes that are actually taken happen to merge harmoniously this aim with the professionals' desire for individual autonomy.

Yet one could argue that a secondary effect of increased and more explicit reporting would be that practices become more open to comparison and external control.[19] In this indirect way, enhancing the objectivity of insurance medicine through increased reporting would still lead us back to the pernicious side effects for the profession's status that we discussed earlier. The transparency that is created through the increased reporting, however, is not without its qualifications. Whereas in many accounts objectivity and transparency are taken to stand for a view "from nowhere" that can see "everywhere,"[20] in this specific case transparency has a quite specific meaning. Rather than implying that the claim evaluation becomes observable and controllable for anyone who cares to look, it becomes quite apparent that there are those who do count as relevant witnesses and those who do not. The reports, first of all, are full of insurance physician jargon and abbreviations. This effectively limits the circle of relevant witnesses to those who are internal to the insurance medicine world—mainly insurance physicians themselves, and perhaps a few outsiders who have learned the jargon.

More important, however, due to the fact that the evaluation process implies a meticulous balancing of a wide array of considerations and information, *the judgment whether this claim evaluation was proper or not requires just as much expert, inside knowledge as the claim evaluation process itself.* The reports are only fully understandable to those who have knowledge of the conventions of the claim evaluation process. They speak of locomotor limitations and psychosocial handicaps, "rest-capacities," and "functional one-armedness." They merge medical jargon with statements that a patient's story is deemed to be consistent with the physical examination, or that the recovery behavior of the client is adequate. For clients, for example, but also for politicians eager to control the rise in disability claims, these reports would be practically meaningless: the only person who can truly grasp and judge these statements is someone with skill and experience comparable to those of the insurance physician themselves. Objectivity, then, implies witnessable, observable, and verifiable *by relevant others*—and those others are quite clearly circumscribed.[21]

Most interviewees stressed the enhanced transparency of the claim evaluation process, while remarking that full transparency would be an impossible goal due to the difficulty and required subtlety of this process. The question *for whom* transparency would be achieved, however, was rarely posed. Only one manager pointed at the highly specific nature of this group of "relevant others." After remarking that standards helped increase transparency, he added that this referred mainly to his role as a manager: he doubted, however, "whether it has become more transparent to the client" (IM). For most interviewees, apparently, their positive evaluation of the achieved transparency has to be seen in the light of the fact that they constitute a small subgroup of all possible witnesses—knowledgeable "insiders"—and that they only consider a small subgroup of possible witnesses as relevant observers—other insiders.

REDEFINING OBJECTIVITY

In his powerful book, *Trust in Numbers*, the historian Porter distinguishes between two types of objectivity that recur throughout the history of the sciences and the histories of accounting, insurance, and public administration. *Disciplinary objectivity* is what typifies powerful, specialist disciplinary communities. Here, consensus is sought and obtained between equals, who comport themselves adequately, are experienced, and are trusted by those requiring their expertise. Disciplinary objectivity is associated with the valuation of tacit knowledge, with the artful application of insight that comes only with learned experience among peers, and with a disdain for standard solutions to complex problems. In the case of *mechanical objectivity*, on the other hand, the trust in experts is replaced by trust in mechanical rules, procedures, and numbers:

> Rules are a check on subjectivity: they should make it impossible for personal biases or preferences to affect the outcome of an investigation. . . . [Mechanical objectivity stands for] a rigorous method, enforced by disciplinary peers, cancelling the biases of the knower and leading ineluctably to valid conclusions. [22]

To understand why the latter form of mechanical, quantitative objectivity has become so dominant throughout the sciences (and public life in general), Porter argues that we should not look to epistemological reasons (such as the higher truth of quantitative objectivity when compared to lesser developed sciences). Nor should we wield the overused rhetoric of ideology (interpreting the claim to objectivity as a mere claim to power). Rather, we have to look at changes in the "social basis of authority" of the expert communities involved. Put briefly, whenever an expert community comes under increased outside pressure—as the medical community in recent years—the legitimacy of personal expertise that typifies disciplinary objectivity erodes, and the expert community is forced to transfer their legitimacy to independently verifiable rules and procedures. When a profession becomes vulnerable, merit shifts from character to method[23]—such as randomized control trials and evidence-based guidelines. Mechanical objectivity, Porter argues, "is a way of making decisions without seeming to decide; [it] lends authority to officials who have very little of their own."[24]

Porter's account reflects interestingly upon the analysis made in this chapter. Insurance medicine is obviously a vulnerable profession, ranking as one of the lowest on the ladder within the medical profession, and under increasing pressure from politicians, employers, and clients alike. Insurance physicians are simultaneously judged in a medical and a legal framework: they are (still) central to the execution of social security laws and have to simultaneously meet medical professional standards. According to Porter's analysis, insurance medicine's turn to guidelines is a prototypical case of the shift from disciplinary to mechanical objectivity. If there was ever a profession in need of external means of legitimacy, it might be this one. And indeed, the insurance physicians we studied were generally quite pleased with the guidelines because they gave them a grip to hold on to, were seen as an acknowledgment of the complexity of their task, and constituted a means to defend their judgments vis-à-vis intruders' opinions and interests.

Yet whereas for Porter disciplinary and mechanical objectivity are exclusive categories (expert communities usually moving from the former to the latter), our analysis suggests that more creative solutions are possible. In the case we studied here, embracing guidelines to support a profession's status did not go hand in hand with a concurrent transfer of decision power from judgment to mechanical rules. Rather than embodying mechanical objectivity, these guidelines seemed to strengthen disciplinary objectivity. The authors and users of the guidelines actively created a space for the weighing of a broad array of diverse elements. The guidelines defined this activity as objective medical evaluation—to be performed and judged only by the qualified members of the profession of insurance physicians.

It is important to stress that this case was not about the accommodation of a space for interpretation and judgment in the guidelines. Most guidelines allow professionals some leeway to deviate from their prescribed path, or to adapt their generic nature to the individual patient.[25] Such an accommodation does not threaten Porter's analysis: such guidelines are still the mechanical framework within which the professional can wield his or her dwindling clinical autonomy. In our case, however, the guidelines did not leave some space but actively created it. They blurred Porter's categories in that they are mechanical tools that have somehow succeeded in strengthening disciplinary objectivity.

Yet not all can be captured in Porter's classification: we might lose sight of the specificity of the insurance physicians' conceptual innovation when we try to fit their objectivity into his categories. We pointed at the interesting alignment between the profession's own interests and their passionate plea for a client-centered approach. Objective claim evaluation implied both weighing carefully diverse considerations and granting a central position to the client. Rather than achieving equity and fair treatment through impartiality and an "impersonal" treatment,[26] objectivity here seems to imply being partial to the client and taking his or her perspective as the starting point for your decision-making process.[27]

In addition, the content of the objectivity that the insurance physicians strove for is not captured in Porter's disciplinary versus mechanical objectivity categorization. The insurance physicians' notion of objectivity aimed explicitly for something much more specific: a symmetrical treatment of medical, psychological, and social issues. The guidelines carefully depict the claim evaluation task as a highly complicated endeavor, whose truth and fairness rest upon an equal and weighed balancing of laboratory tests, the client's psychological profile, and his or her functioning at home and at work.

The redefinition of objectivity undertaken here was not without its internal tensions. We argued that a client-centered approach was a core part of the insurance physician's objective claim evaluation procedure. Yet the specific redefinition of objectivity embedded in these guidelines implied that the claim evaluation reports were transparent only to knowledgeable insiders. Clients, for one, were certainly not included in this category. There are, then, cracks in the alignment between the insurance physicians' professional interests and their aims to acknowledge the patient as responsible, active agent. At the very least, these agents are excluded from fully grasping the decision process that supposedly puts them central stage.

In addition, the transparency achieved through the increased reporting of insurance physicians often ended up being rather opaque. As we saw in Chapter 2, insurance physicians started using standard phrasings on standardized forms to describe claim evaluation cases, which would cover all the necessary legal and professional terminology. This sometimes resulted in long reports that mostly consisted of standard phrases, and that subsequently felt rather empty to those who read the reports. Remarks made about the specific client about whom the report was made had to be carefully looked for in between all the standard sentences. Compared to a brief note, the preset letters seemed to sometimes actually make it harder to get a quick understanding for what exactly the main concern of the specific claim evaluation was.

The specific redefinition of objectivity that the insurance physicians achieved, then, was not without its loose ends. As all definitions, theirs was highly tied to the specific circumstances in which it came about, including the paradoxes and tensions that were inherent in this situation. Amid the overall institutional turmoil in which insurance physicians find themselves, its fate is unclear at this time: the guidelines might not prove a strong enough ally to resist the still existing pressure to be more strict, more clear-cut, and more controllable. They might be contested by policy makers desiring a more unequivocal uniformity in the work of insurance physicians, or by critics within the profession who believe that hard, quantifiable objectivity is the only sure road to professional strength.[28] Whatever its future, however, it now stands as a fascinating example of the attempts of a vulnerable profession to creatively reappropriate objectivity to their own and their clients' ends.

5 Evidence-Based Medicine and Learning to Doctor

BECAUSE EBM centers on information gathering and evaluation, medical educators have suggested an evidence-based curriculum and training to teach students medicine.[1] According to the American Association of Medical Colleges, 88 percent of medical schools in the United States have embraced EBM as a central feature of their curriculum, making it a "quiet educational revolution."[2] Such curricula rest on a simple, yet subversive, principle: instead of relying on how experienced clinicians order them to treat patients, "students of health professions should be encouraged to ask every day, 'What's the evidence?' "[3]

While advocates aim for a more uniform learning environment where the best evidence guides decision making in medical socialization, critics fear instead that EBM will dehumanize care, turning residents into rule-followers preoccupied with legalities and the small steps of guidelines instead of active problem solvers aware of holistic patient care. Drawing on the work of Plato, Brian Hurwitz, for example, provides two reasons for the opinion that medicine based on guidelines is debased: "firstly because guidelines presuppose an average patient rather than the particular patient whom a doctor is endeavouring to treat, and secondly because the knowledge and analysis that go into the creation of guidelines are not rooted in the mental processes of clinicians, but in the minds of guideline developers distant from the consultation."[4] Critics are particularly wary of the inevitable gap between clean, universal research and a messy, localized clinical practice. Although critics evaluate the wave of EBM negatively, they concede that EBM is likely to permeate every nook of medical practice. Yet, the question remains what the actual effects of EBM on medical training are, or even what it means to do EBM.

In the following interview, a medical resident discusses her encounter with her first diabetic patient. This encounter took place in an educational setting that had enthusiastically joined the EBM bandwagon and was meant as an example of doing evidence-based health care.

Int: Could you tell me about a case you had recently that was particularly challenging or rewarding?

Dr. McNair:[5] Let's see. The new onset diabetic child was very interesting because I have never really seen it. He wasn't in for DKA, diabetic ketoacidosis, but he had a very high blood sugar and the parents described the classic history for new onset where he is very thirsty, going to the bathroom a lot, not eating much and not feeling well. It was a very classic history. And the labs, even though he wasn't that advanced a case of DKA, his labs fit nicely with the picture. It was very cool to learn how to manage that kind of patient from the emergency room to settling him in as an in-patient.

Int: How did you know which kind of tests to order?

Dr. McNair: We knew the patient was coming because it was a referral. Because of the nature of diabetes, the child's regular pediatrician knew that he would probably have to be admitted to the hospital for insulin treatment and for a diagnostic work-up. She had done a quick measurement of the blood sugar within her office. We had already a pretty big clue as to he was a diabetic. She called it over. In between the hour or two [before the patient arrived], the senior resident and I in the emergency room read an article in a recent journal about how to manage diabetes.

Int: How did you find that article?

Dr. McNair: We looked it up in MD Consult. There are computers in the ER where you can access a lot of different search programs. I typed "DKA, new onset," and "review." I found an online article in *Contemporary Pediatrics.*

Int: What did the article tell you?

Dr. McNair: It told me a little bit about the pathophysiology of the disease, it gave a really detailed review of when the patient first presents what are likely symptoms, like percentages of certain kind of symptoms and then it went through a very detailed analysis of what kind of work up you should do when they arrive, what sort of emergency treatment you should give and once you get the patient under control, some kind of long-term plan.

Dr. McNair worked in an environment where EBM was strongly encouraged. Yet, from her assessment of the diabetic patient, it is unclear whether the aspiring pediatrician actually applied the principles of EBM. When faced with a new kind of clinical situation—the diagnosis of her first diabetic patient, Dr. McNair relied on a combination of different information tools. The patient came to her attention from the referring physician who had already run a blood sugar test; she then turned to an older resident and together they searched a literature database; they printed out an article that reviewed patient management and used that as a reference point during the patient visit. Does checking a database and printing out a review article amount to the level of evidence required by EBM educators? Such detailed questions about the actual content of medical practice are important because they determine the innovative potential of an EBM curriculum. If EBM is nothing more than checking the computer in addition to asking for information from supervisors, then the scope of educational change is minimal.

In this chapter, we investigate what the flow of EBM means for medical socialization and the acquisition of medical knowledge. The scant preliminary evidence shows that the link between EBM and residency training is not watertight.[6] Although medical students might benefit to a limited degree from an EBM medical curriculum,[7] the immediate demands of residents on the ward seem to make critically appraising the literature before decision making unrealistic.[8] But such findings are based on self-administered questionnaires and do not ask residents about their experience with EBM. Our research is based on in-depth interviews with seventeen pediatric residents of two U.S. pediatric residency programs. Both programs were part of large, urban hospitals affiliated with academic institutions. As residents, our respondents had finished four years of medical school and were at different stages of three years of rotations in different clinical pediatric specialties. Most of the respondents were in their mid-20s and white (three Asian respondents). The gender distribution was nine male and eight female residents. Eight respondents were in their first year of residency, two in the second year, five in the third year, and two chief residents were in their fourth year. Their rotations at the time of the interview varied from the newborn unit, endocrinology, hematology-oncology, pediatric intensive care, pediatric surgery, to the emergency department.[9]

We focus on four topics debated in the literature:

• *What do residents understand under EBM and how relevant is EBM to their daily work?* On the most basic level, EBM refers to the reliance on research-based information in clinical decision making. But even on this basic level the situation lends itself to multiple interpretations.

Modern medicine always has been grounded in laboratory research and clinical observations, so what is new about EBM? An EBM medical practice will differ depending on what kind of research qualifies as evidence and the different clinical situations it pertains to. In order to qualify as EBM, should the resident reserve literature consultations for rare, difficult, and new cases, or especially for routine patient interactions? What literature qualifies as solid evidence, and how should it be read? When can a resident who believes in EBM assume that he or she knows the evidence and skip consulting the literature? We show that, based on the way these questions are answered, there are at least two very different ways of doing EBM in clinical training.

• *How does EBM relate to clinical uncertainty?* Medical sociologists have singled out the management of uncertainty as the key issue facing students learning to doctor. In her landmark article on training for uncertainty, Fox argued that students were overwhelmed by the vast amounts of knowledge to master and the many unknowns in the medical knowledge base.[10] Protocols and other standardized research-based learning tools not only summarize the literature in an easily accessible format but also guide the budding physician through the clinical encounter. Standardized protocols could then be the definitive answer to the problem of clinical uncertainty. In the 2000 edition of *The Handbook of Medical Sociology*,[11] Frederic Hafferty suggests that the rise of EBM might have repercussions for the study of uncertainty. "We might want to revisit the writings of Renée Fox, Donald Light, Jack Haas, and William Shaffir, and others on the nature and impact of uncertainty in medical work and question whether the deployment of protocols and the use of report cards is generating a new definition of uncertainty in medical practice."[12]

• *Does EBM level power differences?* Besides emphasizing more epidemiological-oriented research, EBM advocates envision an egalitarian workplace. The difference between the attending (a supervisor) and the resident (M.D. in specialty training) is not measured in years of experience but in familiarity with the literature and neither has a priori the advantage over the other.[13] "While the experience of 'experts' is still of value, faculty and residents are increasingly expected to base their decision on evidence rather than authority. The resident who in Morning Report answers the question, 'why did you do that?' with 'The attending told me to.' does so at his/her peril. The best role models students see on the clerkship will be faculty and residents who can support their decisions with evidence."[14] Or, "Gone are the days when the seasoned, elder authoritarian clinician was the only one able to make complex decision. Now, with the rules of evidence in hand, even the most novice clinician can enter into complex decision making processes."[15] This democratization impulse is theoretically justified by "adult learning theory or andragogy. According to that theory, learners must understand *why* they need to learn something, take *responsibility* for their learning, exploit their *experience* as a resource, link their *readiness* to learn with the exigency of real-life situations, and orient their learning by *life tasks*."[16] An EBM residency should thus level traditional power hierarchies in favor of critical appraisal skills.

• *How does EBM learning compare to learning by experience?* This question goes to the heart of implementing EBM in clinical practice. At stake is the place of scientific knowledge in health care. While EBM founders take pains to explain that EBM does not stand for simple-minded "cookbook medicine," critics and social observers fear that EBM upsets the precarious balance between science and care. Critics lament that EBM leads to a dehumanization of medical practice.[17] In such exchanges, experience and science are viewed as opposite qualities. We bracket this assumption and investigate instead the extent to which knowledge from experience and scientific research are blurred.

Our purpose in this chapter is thus to investigate empirically the extent to which EBM has altered medical training. In line with the broader position taken in this book, we argue that the actual effects of EBM do not fulfill the doomsday predictions of critics or the increased rationality dreams of evidence supporters. Instead, the political and ontological effects of EBM more subtly change the interrelationship between people (in this case, residents and attending) and their tools of knowledge. Such changes need to be situated in the actual content of clinical decision making, within the daily experience of appropriating and making sense of EBM.

DOING EVIDENCE-BASED MEDICINE

The role of EBM during resident training is defined by where a resident seeks information and how confident he or she feels to act on that information. In most rotations the resident has some autonomy about patient care: he or she is required to diagnose and work up patients, monitor their hospital stay, and order laboratory tests and medications. Since a resident has an M.D. degree and wears the clothes and paraphernalia of a hospital physician, other health care providers and patients expect medical competence.[18] How does EBM feature in the socialization of doctoring?

All residents we interviewed stated that, in Dr. Weiss's words, "the new age of medicine is going toward EBM." The two training programs reflected that trend. They had an active lecture series, and had recently retooled their traditional journal clubs to make them more EBM-friendly. In addition, EBM was recommended by chief residents, supervising attendings, and even pharmaceutical representatives. The latter would try to convince residents to use their drug for new applications while showing them research evidence published in major medical journals (this practice is called "academic detailing"). Certain subspecialties, including newborn nursing, were already heavily protocolized.

Steeped in an EBM-friendly environment, all residents reported that, at least occasionally, they "did" EBM. They agreed that doing EBM implied coming up with the best answer to a clinical diagnostic or treatment question. The best solution entailed patient management that was backed up with recently published research by authorities in the field. EBM offers the resident *a written rationale for patient decisions* and this justification is viewed as an alternative to choosing treatments based on the routines of the attending. Importantly, the respondents sharply bifurcated based on what kinds of literature they considered evidence and what should be done with it. We identified two key orientations to EBM: eleven residents relied on the evidence as *librarians* and six utilized the literature more as *researchers* (see Table 5.1).

Librarian residents expanded the intent of EBM advocates. For the majority of residents, doing EBM meant consulting *any* published resource; the information became authoritative from its text format, the institutional affiliation of its author, and the journal. When asked for an instance of EBM, Dr. Di Maio gave an example of checking the literature for a young patient bit by a parrot. He wondered whether parrot bites warrant special antibiotic treatment. A review article explained that, in contrast to dog bites, no antibiotic treatment is required for avian bites, but that the doctor should check for some typical infections. Although

Table 5.1. Librarian and Researcher Residents' Use of the Literature

	LIBRARIAN RESIDENT	RESEARCHER RESIDENT
Main Characteristic	—*Consulting any* literature	—*Evaluating* research
Evaluation Criteria	—Author, Publication Date, Journal	—Double-Blind Clinical Trials —Statistics
Sources of Evidence	—"Cheat" Books —General Textbooks —Review Articles and Protocols	—Review Articles and Protocols —Primary Research
Focus of Reading	—Abstract, Conclusion	—Methodology, Findings
Database Preference	—M.D. Consult	—M.D. Consult and Others

the article provided Dr. Di Maio with guidance on a topic he did not know much about, it was not based on a systematic review of epidemiological literature.

In line with their broad criteria for EBM, librarian residents relied largely on "cheat books," textbooks, guidelines, and review articles. When asked about sources for EBM, several residents pulled a dog-eared copy of *The Harriet Lane Handbook: A Manual for Pediatric House Officers*[19] out of their pockets. Dr. Abrahams lauded the book as "the bible for pediatric residents." *Harriet Lane* was mainly used to check medication dosages for children, but it also contained a number of elementary protocols on how to treat common ailments. In a pinch, residents could quickly glance over such protocols or double-check their initial ideas. The next lines of defense for librarians were the thick, general textbooks that are strewn over the different pediatric wards. The 600-plus-page *Manual of Pediatric Therapeutics*,[20] for example, provides a basic orientation on how to handle most common disorders with some general explanation, but it is less up-to-date and comprehensive than some of the other sources. Because residents have consulted those or similar textbooks throughout medical school, they are familiar with their organization and know that a textbook can "get them by." The most sophisticated literature sources consulted by librarians consisted of protocols provided by professional organizations such as the American Academy of Pediatrics.[21] On a similar level were review articles published in leading pediatric journals that critically assessed the state of the field and the strength of the evidence. When reading such articles, librarians skimmed the methodology and focused on the conclusion and research findings.

Librarians found much evidence via the database MD Consult.[22] This user-friendly database offered the advantage of providing full-text, on-line accessibility and was also linked to some major textbooks. The database avoided a trip to the library. Dr. Weiss noted that the library "is about a five-minute walk. It is on the opposite side of the hospital. So, it is not very convenient." The core of EBM for librarian residents was the pragmatic reliance on literature to solve quickly the dilemma at hand. For that reason, librarians thought that medicine had always been steeped in EBM. Dr. Cole noted, "I think it is like a new term for what medicine is and always has been: using the literature to come up with the best intervention. It is just that things have gotten sloppy, in that people are just going off their own experience and not using the literature to look critically. I feel like this new movement is a reinstitution of this whole idea."

In contrast to the residents who used the literature as librarians, a minority of residents took the core of EBM to mean that the physician acted more as a researcher who actively evaluates and interprets the literature. Residents who professed to be more familiar with EBM specified that merely checking published literature is insufficient but that EBM implies a critical assessment of available evidence in a meta-analysis. Ideally, recommended treatments should have been tested and then replicated in large, prospective, randomized, double-blind, controlled clinical trials by authorities in the field. For researcher residents, the persuasive strength of recommendations does not depend on where findings are published. Two doctors pointed out that the authoritative American Academy of Pediatrics regularly publishes guidelines that are not backed up with statistical evidence but only express the consensus of experts in the field. Such recommendations merely take the problem of basing medicine on routines to a professional level. Researchers use protocols and review articles as an intermediary step to more specialized evidence.

Researcher residents would not consider the parrot bite literature search an instance of EBM. Because of small numbers, the evidence of rare conditions did not meet epidemiological norms but remained necessarily anecdotal. For researcher users of EBM, statistical criteria provided a gold standard for evaluating recommendations. Applying statistical measures makes it possible to make very fine distinctions between studies. Researchers did not look in the scientific literature for pragmatic guidance to treat the patient at hand, but for a variety of factors to take into consideration during decision making. Besides MD Consult, researcher residents also used other databases, such as PubMed, Grateful Med, OVID, the Cochrane library, or Medline. Those sources might provide a more complete overview of a topic, but required an extra trip to the library.

In sum, pediatric residents in both programs reported that the use of evidence was actively encouraged and positively valued and that their involvement in EBM was inevitable. Yet, they defined EBM flexibly to match their own work approaches. From the much quoted EBM definition as "the conscientious, explicit, and judicious use of current best evidence in making decisions about the care of individual patients,"[23] librarians highlighted the practice of checking the literature when diagnostic or treatment problems arose. Researcher residents emphasized the scientific evaluation of research but they questioned the value of EBM's main instruments: guidelines and protocols. Researchers considered EBM a new epidemiology-infused paradigm for medicine. Residents define EBM thus in two different ways and those varying definitions help explain how they appreciate EBM's potential to reduce the uncertainty of a clinical knowledge base.

UNCERTAINTY AND EVIDENCE-BASED MEDICINE

The concept of uncertainty plays a central role in medical sociology scholarship to address the question of how medical knowledge is acquired.[24] Based on research in Cornell's medical school during the early 1950s, Renée Fox argued that medical knowledge is inherently uncertain because it is riddled with gaps and unknowns and, second, because the amount of medical facts is ever-expanding and impossible to master completely.[25] The dilemma for students in medical school consists of managing the limitations of their own cognitive ability and the vast medical literature. During residents' clinical years, medical uncertainty emerges when students apply text knowledge to clinical situations and handle both the physiological and psychological aspects of patient care. Fox's sociology of knowledge consists of a gradual socialization in medical confidence; instead of blaming oneself for clinical mistakes, the aspiring doctor learns to manage successfully the limitations of medicine. In later writings, Fox argued that uncertainty has become the hallmark of the entire field of medicine.[26]

Other authors have questioned the primacy of uncertainty and instead highlighted that training for uncertainty is closely followed by training for control.[27] Based on fieldwork among psychiatrists during their residency years, Donald Light proposed that the goal of medical training is to teach young physicians how to control their uncertainties in order to become professional experts within their field.[28] Instead of being imbued with scientific skepticism, Atkinson portrays medical students as pragmatists, "content to work within the conceptual bounds of a given 'paradigm.'"[29] Following Alfred Schutz, Atkinson argues that certainty and uncertainty are two different phenomenological attitudes of the same medical discourse, reflecting different practical and theoretical interests. Only emphasizing uncertainty downplays medicine's dogmatic character. Finally, psychiatrist Jay Katz also argued that, propelled by uncertainty, the pendulum can swing too far in the opposite direction.[30] The mechanisms that physicians learn for coping with uncertainty lead them to disregard and avoid uncertainty.

While most sociologists—and also most medical practitioners—agree that the medical knowledge base is marred by various uncertainties, scholarly disagreements persist on the dominance of uncertainty and on whether uncertainty and certainty imply each other. Because EBM relies on a standardization of medical knowledge and technique, it can be seen as a catalyst for these opposing viewpoints.[31] In her most recent update of the uncertainty literature, Fox addresses the surge of EBM. Fox contends that EBM reinforces collective-oriented approaches in medicine at the expense of individualized patient-doctor interactions.[32] Siding with the critics of EBM, Fox remains apprehensive of EBM's narrow empiricist positivism and its threat to clinical expertise. Fox does not address the way EBM would impact medical socialization but, based on the central message of her earlier work, we would expect that the rise of EBM perpetuates an attitude of scientific skepticism.

EBM would help students "achieve as much cognitive command of the situation as possible. . . . [Students] became more able to accept uncertainty as inherent in medicine, to sort out their own limitations from those of the field, meet uncertainty with candor, and to take a 'positive, philosophy-of-doubting' approach."[33]

With Light, Katz, and Atkinson we would expect that EBM perpetuates a dogmatic, control-centered form of medicine in residents' daily clinical practice, validating the power of medicine while accentuating the strengths and weaknesses of its scientific basis. Light, for example, notes that emphasizing technique serves as a major form of professional control, providing a technical understanding of competence.

The residents we interviewed, however, noted that the most immediate effect of the increased reliance on guidelines and medical literature was a new source of uncertainty to be managed. Residents not only need to know how to diagnose and treat patients but how to acquire epidemiological research skills as well. Research-based uncertainty deals with the actual practice of conducting literature searches and evaluating studies.[34] Even residents who rarely consulted primary research acknowledged that such critical assessment skills were expected of them. We found three instances of this novel uncertainty.

First, some residents felt uncomfortable about their ability to search for primary or review articles. Their concerns were focused on their knowledge about how to navigate effectively the computer search engines. To conduct a good search, residents had to know which search engines existed, what kinds of information each source held, and how to search each one with appropriate "key terms." Dr. Cole described the difficulty he encountered when trying to master new search engines. "They [the library] also have a number of other evidence-based programs that I am not even so familiar with yet, like the Cochrane database and Best Evidence. I have tried to use them, but I haven't really learned how to use them. They are not so easy to just log-on and use. I have tried to just throw in a couple of terms, thinking it would be self-evident how it worked. It wasn't."

Second, residents expressed their discomfort in evaluating the quality of primary articles. Librarians and researcher residents expressed similar doubts about their abilities to evaluate an article effectively. Even Dr. Mouton, who had worked for several years in biomedical research, acknowledged that she was "not a very good statistician." Other residents who had taken courses in medical school in biostatistics or epidemiology still felt unsure about their abilities to distinguish between a good sample and a bad sample, and statistical significance and confidence intervals. Dr. McNair expressed her confusion. "I know the word is to power a study but I have no idea how to calculate that. I know you reach a statistical significance that is accepted in clinical medicine where the p value is less than 0.05 you assume that there is less than a 5 percent chance that the results are due to chance alone. That is pretty much the extent of my statistics."

Third, residents questioned the rationale behind conducting studies and expressed suspicion about the effects of economical incentives on the quality of medical knowledge. Dr. Weiss noted that "studies follow money, where money is, will be many studies. But at the same time, no one is going to do research on common things that we don't have any questions about." Similarly, Dr. Brown remarked that she tends to be skeptical of the sources of research funding, "I always look at the source: who did the study, was it a pharmaceutical company or were, the authors supported by them. They have to disclose that." The circulation of money and prestige leads to an imbalance in the availability of evidence: some diseases and conditions will receive more attention (a resident pointed out the cardiovascular bias in medicine) while others might be neglected. The available research funding might thus sway the entire medical field. Pediatricians were particularly attuned to this inequity because comparatively little research exists on treatments and drug dosages for children.

The new research-based uncertainty leads to new forms of managing the uncertainty. Chief residents and attendings would organize journal clubs where residents presented and critiqued articles, offered statistics refresher courses, and gave tutorials on how to use Medline effectively. Guest speakers would tour departments and lecture on the primary research they had conducted. And consistent with the spirit of EBM, medical journals would publish literature guidelines. Learning how to deal with the specific uncertainty of research led, thus, to a new kind of research-infused skill, an additional dimension of learning to doctor.

The important issue at stake is the net result of the infusion of EBM for clinical practice: do residents display an attitude of scientific doubting as Fox predicted, or does EBM confirm medical dogmatism, as Atkinson, Katz, and Light feared? The answer to that question depends on the different research approaches of librarian and researcher residents toward the different sources of EBM. In short, librarians act more along the lines set out by Atkinson, Katz, and Light while researchers follow Fox's predictions (see Table 5.2).

For librarian residents, practicing EBM with guidelines and review articles provided some comfort within the chaos of their clinical training. Residents suggested that a literature search allowed them to orient themselves when they had a diagnostic or a treatment question. They used the literature to make sure they were in the ballpark before addressing the attending or their colleagues about a patient. Dr. Cole gave an example of how EBM reduces clinical uncertainty. He talked about a patient with abnormal lab results, possibly indicating hepatitis or myositis:

> People are still calling it a hepatitis/myositis, but I think that the only reason we are calling it a hepatitis is because some of her liver function tests are abnormal, but it is only some of them and, it is the ones that could be elevated in skeletal-muscle disease. I think it is just going to be obvious to everyone when I tell them this afternoon. It has sort of been thrown around but no one has said for sure. But now, I have these papers that say the [test results] can go up with skeletal-muscle disease. Boom! Now when I take it to them, I am more confident in my diagnosis.

Table 5.2.   Residents and the Management of Uncertainty

	Librarian Resident	Researcher Resident
Guidelines and Protocols	—Comfortable, Authoritative —Legal Protection	—False Sense of Security
Clinical Trials	—Insufficiently Directive	—Render Decisions Complex
Consequence for Medical Practice	—Follow Guidelines —Avoid Research	—Disregard Guidelines —Interpret Research
Applying EBM in general	—Too Standardized to Qualify as "Real Medicine"	—"Real Medicine" Supposes Understanding Uncertainty
Uncertainty Attitude	—Tendency to Dogmatism	—Tendency to Skepticism

Here, the literature boosted Dr. Cole's hunches. To find this type of comfort, however, librarian residents tended to search prepackaged EBM: review articles and guidelines where experts in the field had already sorted through the evidence. Dr. McNair commented how a review article helped her determine the typical treatment for a diabetic child. "I know a lot of pathophysiology, but I don't know how to do the work-up and treat the child. I use a lot of articles, especially review articles, large group studies, to figure out what my steps should be."

Librarian residents mentioned that guidelines provided an additional kind of legal comfort that has become more accentuated recently in North American health care. Following a guideline approved by the American Academy of Pediatrics might provide some protection from malpractice lawsuits. Dr. McDougall explained the benefit. "You always have clinical liability on your side. I follow the guidelines that the AAP has set. They can't fault you when you have done everything you can for that person." In contrast, consulting clinical trials might present legal pitfalls. Dr. Tomassi warned, "A lot of times the primary literature is very much like 'well, some studies suggest this, some studies suggest that' and then you don't know what the hell to do with this. Do I want to do anything because I read in an article that I am not familiar with? Will that get me sued or kill a patient because just some study told me so?"

Researcher residents, however, were hesitant about using the authority of guidelines to make themselves feel more comfortable or to meet legal protections. Dr. Mouton suggested that guidelines might make residents feel too complacent. "One of the things that I think is wrong is if you go into medical school and grasp whatever bit of guidelines you can get to cover your insecurities. If you do that then you stop thinking. That is probably the biggest pitfall of guidelines. People stop using their common sense. [A guideline] doesn't mean that you shouldn't examine the baby." To avoid a false sense of security, researchers tended to question critically the directives of guidelines and review articles instead of taking it as medical gospel.

With clinical trials and other forms of primary research, the opinions ran opposite. Librarian residents remarked that primary studies inevitably generated contradictions and confusions. Dr. Fletcher stressed her frustration. "This is probably a little too honest. But you spend all this time reading that stinking study and then you come up with one thing at the very end. The result was maybe this or maybe that. And sometimes it is equivocal. (She throws up her arms.) I just want to know what is done. What is the result? And typically the thing you pull is not even the question you are asking." Dr. Mouton, more of a researcher resident, stressed instead that the contradictions revealed in primary research do not necessarily lead to worse clinical practice. She stated:

> It is very hard to find certain truths. The literature doesn't help you to find those kinds of securities. The literature makes you aware of all the little edges. When you go to the literature you always find something that makes you think: "Oh, I shouldn't forget that" or "Oh, I should think about this." When you do a literature search it makes you more knowledgeable. Being more knowledgeable makes you more certain where you stand.

While for librarian residents the primary literature perpetuated confusion and led to an avoidance of such studies, researcher residents acknowledged the conflicting picture of different studies but stressed—in Dr. Mouton's words—that "controversy is part of life, part of research, part of science." Primary research alerted researcher residents to factors and variations of clinical practice that they should not take for granted. The result was a more complex decision-making process in which uncertainties within medical knowledge were incorporated.

When applying EBM to clinical dilemmas they face in their practice, librarian and researcher residents were again at odds about the merits of evidence. For librarian residents, any literature was fundamentally incomplete. Dr. Tomassi put the problem simply: "Guidelines cannot diagnose the patient for me." Librarians reacted against the widespread stereotype that EBM would take the place of clinical judgment, reducing them to mere short-order cooks who followed "cookbook-recipe" medicine. Librarian residents pointed out that EBM only touched on the real work of managing patients and could never take the place of clinical judgment. Dr. McNair noted that the problem with EBM lies exactly in its standardization. "Not everyone fits into these nice little boxes where you can just label them and do this, and this, and you should have this happen."

For librarian residents, the ultimate litmus test of reducing uncertainty and gaining certitude is having done things repeatedly in the past. Whether such tried practice was grounded in the attending's standard of care or in the literature did not matter much. Because the attending's advice was likely to be tailored to the individual patient's situation, it might have an edge for residents in training. A resident noted that he seemed to get clinical results, regardless of the source he used. And if he did not obtain expected results, he would try something different next time. The basic issue was not to kill patients and not to get sued. This philosophy led librarian residents to avoid doing too many literature searches.

Researcher residents were also aware of the gap between the literature and clinical practice in the immediate pressures of residency life. Dr. Weiss articulated the tensions: "The limitations [of EBM] are that it is tough to access unless you have the time to do it all the time . . . unless you are really up on the literature. It is kind of like surfing. Once you are on the board and going down the wave it is easy; but you have to paddle and get up on the board first. I guess as a resident you are too busy just trying to make sure the board doesn't come crashing down on you to do that."

But where librarian residents considered literature searches, at best, a dubious tool for reducing clinical uncertainty and more commonly a source of extra frustration, researcher residents embraced dealing with the contradictions and confounding variables of both patient care and the literature as real medical work. Teasing out protocols and research findings was as important as managing a blood pressure. One of the surprising findings in our interviews was that the clinical examples provided by the most EBM-knowledgeable residents centered around disregarding research, adapting protocols and guidelines, or filling gaps in the literature. Researcher residents argued that EBM might lead to better physicians who know when *not* to follow research-based guidelines and recommendations.

In conclusion, librarian residents look to the research literature for ready answers but are disappointed with the uncertainty inherent in medical knowledge. Researcher residents, on the other hand, trust that uncertainty produced by the literature and clinical practice creates a positive flux of increased knowledge. Librarians' instrumentalist use of the literature is more likely to confirm a dogmatic clinical practice. Librarian residents might overstate the certainty of research and take recommendations at face value, or—more commonly—they might get frustrated with the residual uncertainty of research findings and avoid researching altogether. Researcher residents approach the literature from a more relativist perspective. They do not expect clear answers but a sharpening of discriminatory power that will aid them in patient decision making. Researcher residents apply the critical assessment skills touted by EBM advocates to EBM itself, leading to a skeptical research attitude and disregarding of EBM. Fox's analysis seems thus to be more geared toward a minority group of researcher residents who adopt uncertainty as their clinical leitmotiv while Atkinson, Katz, and Light quite accurately predicted the attitude of librarian residents for whom the urge to dominate clinical uncertainty with ready-made knowledge prevails. Both librarian and resident residents do not apply an a priori notion of "clinical judgment," but they rely on different resources (textbooks and own research) to develop an appropriate clinical practice.

LEVELING OF POWER DIFFERENCES

When new residents enter the Department of Obstetrics, Gynecology, and Reproductive Sciences of San Francisco General Hospital, they receive a written manifesto about evidence-based medicine. "The manifesto levels the intellectual playing field: Everyone's clinical opinion counts equally, regardless of rank or experience. We value opinions only to the extent that they are supported by scientific evidence, and not according to the perceived prestige of the proponent."[35] This manifesto is only the most explicit instance of a general assumption that evidence serves as the great power equalizer.[36] Access to the research literature is supposed to break down the experience advantage of attendings and lead to a leveling of the clinical field.[37] Instead of reaching decisions on what has been the tradition in a hospital or on what their superiors tell them to do, residents need to become critical researchers who chart their own treatment plans based on the research literature. The authority of medicine shifts from whoever happens to be the attending on call to the true experts in the broader field of pediatrics.

Did the residents experience the benefits of democratization in an EBM-friendly environment? Our residents reported that EBM has not resulted in complete egalitarianism. The reality of the pediatric residency training is that most residents only in emergency situations decide upon their own treatments without previously consulting a senior resident or an attending. Like Dr. McNair's work-up of the diabetic patient, they almost always run their ideas by a senior. Residents admitted to only settling on laboratory tests on their own if they had previously seen several similar patients. Sociologist Charles Bosk has noted that attendings also consult with colleagues to diminish uncertainty,[38] but the difference is that residents are required to always consult. Even when one of the programs billed its relationship between residents and attendings as collegial teamwork, the residents understood that they were at the bottom of a steep hierarchy.

Almost every resident, including third years and the chief residents, confirmed their marginal status. Dr. Mouton acknowledged that she was "the lowest on the whole ladder here." Dr. Chambliss added, "I don't feel like I am on the same level with anybody right now." And Dr. Rosenberg noted that the inequality was actually beneficial to the resident. "Frankly, as a resident I think it is a treat for it not to be a level playing field. They have the experience and are comfortable making decisions. They know what to do. We are still learning. We don't know what to do half of the time. And I am not saying this in a complacent kind of a way. But, the pressure is not so much on us." Within such a supervisory apprenticeship, the aim of residency is to build a foundation in a variety of pediatric cases. Dr. Weiss explained, "The idea of residency is to get in there first, find out what your gut feeling is, what you think it is, and then present it to somebody else and bounce it off them. They will say, 'I disagree with this. You forgot this. You might want to look into this.'" Almost all examples of medical decision making included checking ideas with experienced senior residents or attendings.[39]

Because residents reside at the bottom of a steep authority ladder, few residents actively challenged attendings or pointed out that their superiors' recommendations were outdated when their own critical literature and research review suggested alternative patient management. At best they might engage in a polite, face-saving discussion about what might be most beneficial for the patient or ask the attendings what they thought of a particular alternative. Even in such exchanges, most residents reported that they and the literature would likely lose out. Dr. Wilson noted that "at those times it tends to fall back on experience. [The attending would say:] 'well, that may work, but I have seen in this case, this works better. So we are going this way.'" The attending would qualify the study's findings with some reason why the recommendations did not apply in this particular case.[40]

Dr. Mouton added a classic authority-based argument to explain her lack of confrontation. "I think I rely more on the guidelines and that is just because I am an employee of this system and they have the guidelines. I make my superiors happier and make my own life much easier if I just stick with guidelines." Dr. Chambliss also reported that even if he knew an attending was wrong, he was unlikely to point it out because "the pecking order is unfortunately well established." Residents noted that they were unlikely to know as much about the patient or the literature, and that they lacked the thirty years of experience to engage in a discussion among equals. Even considering the research literature, they did not think that they had enough time to read through articles, absorb the material, retain it, and apply it on a daily basis. The attending was not only likely to have more experience with patients, but also might know the reputation of a particular hospital for orthopedics, the extent to which a particular author opts for "unnecessary" tests, or the kind of publishing criteria used in a journal.

Not only did residents confirm that their superiors' institutionalized power advantage and accumulated experience trumped any knowledge they might have gleaned from the literature, but they also admitted that they would act similarly when others challenged them. We asked how residents would react if medical students (even lower in the hierarchy) questioned residents' treatment of choice with research-based evidence. Their answer revealed a pattern similar to the one they were subjected to: listen politely, and evaluate whether the evidence might be relevant if time permits, but "likely stick with experience."

Despite the lack of total democratization with science, EBM impacted the relationship between attendings and residents because it restructured the knowledge exchange. EBM offered residents and attendings an external baseline from which to evaluate the knowledge base of the other. Most attendings are not keepers of outdated traditions but instead "guarantors" of EBM usage, ensuring continuous reminders and consistency.[41] EBM became integrated in a hierarchical relationship where superiors asked residents to conduct literature searches when questions arose. Dr. Wilson explained, "It is not uncommon to have your attending ask you, 'Why don't you check that out?' or 'Why don't you see if you can find some information about that?'" In turn, senior residents asked younger residents to find out, for example, the latest about a new generation of antibiotics. Once the resident comes up with the most recent literature, attendings might sit down with them and discuss the strengths and weaknesses of the evidence. Dr. Weiss speculated that many attendings liked working with residents because they have an opportunity to learn from them. "That is why certain attendings stick around university settings, because they want to feed off residents."

The literature can also be used as a benchmark to evaluate the competency of an attending. Several residents mentioned that they checked up on their attending while comparing the latter's standard treatments with what the literature recommended. Dr. Gross stated, "I usually look up articles so I can understand where they (attendings) are coming from, to see if what they say agrees with the articles or not. If it doesn't at all, then I would probably ask another attending." Besides specialization and general approachability ("we don't go to the big scary attending"), residents called upon attendings who admitted their own knowledge gaps and encouraged residents to check the literature. Valued attendings were open-minded about different treatment options, but were also able to reach clinical decisions. Dr. McNair explained, "I use how many years of experience they have, how competent they seem in their answer, and whether or not they seem well versed in the literature or their field."

When residents encounter a dilemma or new situation, a literature review allows them to channel their ignorance before they approach the attending. Dr. Weiss put it this way: "Guidelines, for residents, ensure that you are not totally in left field. It gives you a chance of not missing something that you shouldn't have missed, but you don't have the experience to know that yet. So, it buys you somebody else's experience, I guess." The protocols and research recommendations gave the resident a hunch of what this patient might be all about, but whether clues translated into realities depended on whether the attending would go along with the recommendations or instead suggest alternatives. As Dr. Cole explained, it is often simpler and easier to ask than to research. "A more efficient way is to reach for help. In the times that I do have to research, it is great. You find out how much information there is. Then, when you go to speak with the attendings, you realize that they generally know, broadly, what the issues are and what the best treatment is.

But, the particulars they don't always know. They can't." Occasionally, the literature also offered the resident an alternative to interacting directly with an unpopular attending. Research allowed residents to "get by and bystep" attendings.

Attendings and residents who take EBM's democratization promise seriously are thus in for a rude awakening. Residents overwhelmingly acknowledged that even with guidelines and protocols hierarchy differences are real and cannot be ignored. Attendings function not only as more experienced colleagues but also as supervisors whose evaluations carry much weight. Even in a medical world in which protocols and guidelines spell out best practices, residents still need to decipher—in Dr. Chambliss's words—"the attending's best practice." Written knowledge cannot overcome the barrier of accumulated experience and pedagogical supervision. Residents differentiate between what the attendings expect them to do and what they hope to do once they work on their own. Pleasing the attending was an extra skill to acquire when learning to doctor.[42] This skill might or might not overlap with what the literature recommends. EBM does thus not invert power relationships but is seamlessly integrated in existing pedagogical authority differences.

This does not mean that EBM has no political effects in medical training. EBM might not take away the uncertainty of medical socialization but it alters the attending-resident relationship in more indirect and subtle ways. EBM in general has shifted the direction of medicine from pathophysiological observations to epidemiological studies based on clinical trials.[43] As such, the body of medical knowledge is not necessarily more transparent but more accessible. The rise of information technologies and specialized databases provides quick access to the literature from most patient wards and clinics. Within the context of the resident-attending relationship, EBM forms an external validation criterion for both resident and attending to check the other's knowledge base. Residents consult the literature to impress attendings, and they in turn impress their charges with references to studies and clinical practice guidelines. Once residents master the intricacies of EBM, they can channel their uncertainty before facing the attending. In light of these changes, Dr. Rosenberg granted that instead of leveling the playing field, EBM "brings the field a little bit closer."

THE FRONTIER OF CLINICAL JUDGMENT

Wherever we turn, the formal tools of EBM seem to run into a barrier of clinical judgment and experience. Research-based knowledge seems to perpetually fall short in clinical decision making. Residents refer to the extra quality needed as "experience," "competence," or "confidence." Even EBM advocates add the caveat that EBM should never be interpreted as a substitute for clinical judgment.[44] Sociologists seem to agree with medical practitioners when they stress that control over uncertainty is achieved with a growing sense of confidence. Concepts such as confidence, certitude, and experience are crucial in socialization theory, but they remain difficult to articulate and most sociologists attribute experience simply to the resident's seniority.[45] After some time, the resident somehow has acquired experience and gained confidence. Part of the conceptual difficulty is that experience and evidence continue to be viewed as distinct, even opposite, entities.

Residents' encounters with EBM show that pure "informal experience" and "formal evidence" do not really exist. Any consultation of written research is already prestructured by the overall diagnostic or treatment goal and informed by other research and accumulated clinical observations. Similarly, any experience is grounded in the hierarchy of written research evidence, anecdotes, consensus, and hunches of generations of clinicians and basic researchers. "Evidence" and "experience" constitute complementary resources that help residents in learning treatment options and patient management.[46] The point of EBM in residency training is not to impose simplistic rule following but to offer a justification for clinical decision making. As we have seen in Chapter 2, in order to make practice guidelines work, residents need to submit actively to the prescriptions of the standards. Librarians will check ready-made evidence while researchers are more likely to assess primary literature. But those findings are filtered through the attending who, in turn, has accumulated an amalgam of patient experiences and research findings. The quality that guides clinical decision making is not the tradition-bound experience put up as a straw person in the medical and sociological literature, but a mixture of skills and uncertainties grounded in medical knowledge.

Medical knowledge acquisition can thus not be reduced to either evidence or experience but inevitably contains a mixture of the two, albeit not necessarily in equal proportions. Librarians as a group tend to prefer the hands-on handling of patients and the visual instruction of attendings while researcher residents ground their expertise in the literature. But librarians still need to acquire evidence to back up their practice while researchers must fall back on hands-on patient handling to decide how the literature applies. Second, residents with good medical knowledge skills do not necessarily use more literature but exhibit an awareness of all the factors necessary to reach a satisfactory medical decision. A competent resident knows when literature reviews will likely lead to better patient care, how to evaluate research findings effectively, how to check the findings with the attending in a way that preserves the senior's authority, and how to communicate the proposed decision plan with the patient to ensure adequate compliance. Evidence-based clinical judgment thus includes epidemiological and social skills.

Although rooted in research and literature, the medical knowledge acquisition process moves the resident away from a strict interpretation of the literature. A physician starts with a recommendation and adds qualifications to consider whether the guideline applies to this particular patient, ward, attending, time frame, and resources. The generation of clinical judgment allows residents to apply protocols to patients for whom it was not intended because they gained insights into the rationale behind the evidence. It also facilitates skipping or substituting steps, working around the protocols, and appropriating them. The resident interacts with the protocols and guidelines. More than the mere passing of time, the relative value of factors to be taken into consideration marks the accumulation of medical knowledge.

The legacy of introducing evidence-based medicine in residency training rests thus in the subtle honing of a critical awareness when learning the tricks of the medical trade. The practical development of this particular kind of clinical judgment is largely unrelated to the intentions of EBM proponents or the fears of its critics. Supporters offer EBM as a solution to the problem of variability while critics fear that standardization leads to dehumanization of care. Critics and supporters view EBM as a clear and straightforward plan of action authorized by scientific imperative. Instead, EBM accentuates some of the messy contradictions of medicine for residents. They learn that medicine is scientifically grounded but its scientific base is also riddled with unknowns and uncertainties, that large critical clinical trials are superior sources of knowledge but rarely provide conclusive answers, and that variation in clinical practice should be avoided although different treatments seem to be equally helpful in caring for patients. The proposed problem for which EBM is the solution does not match the reality of learning to doctor. Residents generally do not agonize as much about variability or dehumanizing care as they worry about getting through the residency without killing patients, completely exhausting themselves, accumulating negative evaluations, or getting sued.

The issue is not to use EBM in clinical decision making for the sake of science but, more pragmatically, to figure out what kind of evidence might be appropriate in dealing with patients. Good clinical practice does not demand saturation with EBM but results in a wide range of kinds of evidence that might be applied at varying times with different consequences. The determining factor in a resident's learning process is the level of uncertainty he or she is comfortable handling in decision making. The paradox of learning with standards is that more EBM actually generates more uncertainty, less EBM often leads to a clearer practice. Similarly, in these educational settings, EBM did not erase preexisting unequal power relationships but introduced information technologies and epidemiological criteria in the personal dynamic. Both groups could use these new tools to leverage the situation. The result was that EBM erased some previous power disadvantages (attendings traditionally had better access to the research literature and follow-up information)[47] and at the same time perpetuated other power components (attendings usually still remain more familiar with the literature).

6 Standardizing Risk
A Case Study of Thalidomide

THE U.S. Food and Drug Administration (FDA) and the drug company Celgene faced a complicated and sensitive issue in the late 1990s, when they intended to introduce the drug thalidomide to the U.S. market. Currently, the drug is recognized as a promising treatment for a virtually endless list of serious, life-threatening diseases, including AIDS wasting syndrome.[1] But thalidomide has a dark and dangerous past: it was promoted in the late 1950s as a sedative and treatment for morning sickness (under different brand names; e.g., Distaval and Softenon), before scientists and physicians discovered that it caused neurotoxicity among some patients and devastating congenital malformations among babies born to women who took the drug while they were pregnant. The babies had stunted, flipper-like extremities with missing fingers or limbs. The problem with marketing thalidomide in the new millennium is not just the drug's well-documented toxicity (many drugs on the market are just as toxic, if not more so), but also its deep symbolic value. Thalidomide played a key role in shaping U.S. drug regulation. After thousands of babies were born with congenital malformations worldwide and the disaster barely missed the United States, a stringent drug regulation bill that had been lingering in congressional committees quickly became legislation. Thalidomide and the malformed babies symbolized the horror of unregulated drugs.

Thalidomide's relationship with evidence-based medicine is manifold. As briefly alluded to in Chapter 3, it was the worldwide thalidomide disaster that triggered tighter FDA regulations and required drug manufacturers to prove the efficacy and safety of the drugs they intended to bring to market. These new regulations institutionalized the randomized clinical trial as the scientific gold standard in health care, in turn providing the preferred raw material for evidence-based medicine evaluations. As part of the drug approval process, drug manufac-

166

turers, including Celgene,[2] have to prove that their drug outperforms placebos in trials on human subjects (phase 2 and 3 clinical trials). At a later stage, these clinical trials in combination with other independent studies contribute to the evidence of a clinical practice guideline aimed at practitioners to discuss the appropriate prescription of the drug.

The thalidomide case study thus provides an entrance into one of the most standardized areas of contemporary health care: drug approval and prescription. Drug manufacturers have been strategic supporters of evidence-based medicine. They have particularly supported the dissemination of clinical guidelines that established the superiority of their drug—which they of course fund, generating another manifestation of a seamless medical-industrial complex.[3] They have reached out to individual clinicians, professional organizations, pharmacists, patient groups, and government regulators to disseminate the positive results of clinical trials, aiming for "evidence-based pharmacotherapy."[4] While providing some of the funding and other resources for clinical practice guidelines, drug manufacturers have also flooded the market with drug promotions and marketing strategies that only occasionally rely on scientific evidence.[5] The result is a skewing of medical knowledge in favor of drug therapies, contributing to the great variability of drug prescription among geographic areas.[6] A study of the treatment of osteoarthritis of the knee joint showed, for example, that the available evidence was dominated by studies of pharmaceutical and surgical interventions while consumers and primary clinicians expressed greater interest in alternative forms of treatment (including life-style changes and education).[7]

The distribution of risk is also an issue in all clinical practice guidelines.[8] Every guideline evaluating an intervention or therapy implicitly or explicitly determines whether the benefits of treatment outweigh the risk of treatment and nontreatment.[9] Yet, in the construction of the thalidomide distribution system the stakes of risk were particularly high. The drug could prove beneficial, even life-saving, to a great number of patients, but distributing the risk to the "wrong" persons could cause severe disabilities and could even result in a major public relations disaster for drug regulators and the pharmaceutical industry.

This chapter provides a detailed analysis of how exactly risk is perceived, located, and neutralized in the context of standardization. In addition, an analysis of standards in the making provides insights in how physicians articulate their professional roles and responsibilities. As we have seen in previous chapters, a great impetus for standardization is pressure from external parties to hold health care providers accountable. Regulatory meetings where procedural standards are formulated constitute the battlegrounds where third parties propose to advance on or confirm professional autonomy. This chapter also provides insight into the claims and priorities of parties that have remained more in the background in other chapters, such as patients, drug regulators, and pharmacists. By focusing on how these different parties approach standardization of their own and each other's jurisdiction, we highlight these political rearrangements in the design phase, before standards are put into place. During the designing process, crucial decisions are made about the leeway each set of actors has in the proposed system. If the standard is successful in rendering behavior uniform over time and across geographical areas, those decisions are quickly forgotten or taken for granted. A review of a standard in the making provides information about how choices are made and which political alliances the standard will need to foster. Importantly, a look over the designers' shoulders brackets the ingrained assumptions about power differences and indicates how "it could have been different."[10]

Distributing thalidomide in the United States pits the risk of congenitally malformed babies against the promise of treating life-threatening conditions. We argue that the standardized distribution system, through defining risk in a specific way, consolidated important normative choices. During the debates about the distribution system, risk emerges as a quality that is unequally distributed among participants. The standardized distribution system made the risk for congenital malformations acceptable (it *normalized* risk), through locating the danger for a new generation of thalidomide babies with particular groups while minimizing the responsibility of other groups. The classic example of the normalization of risk is Diane Vaughan's in-depth analysis of the disastrous launching of the space shuttle, the *Challenger*.[11] Poring over transcripts and interviews, Vaughan shows how previously unacceptable engineering and safety criteria were redefined to acceptable—and thus launchable—measures. In the case of thalidomide, the standardized thalidomide distribution system was put in place to control the risk of this drug. It altered the perception of the risk of congenital malformation to such an extent that most actors were willing to sign on to the distribution system. The risk that previously seemed insurmountable became acceptable through the new distribution system, which coordinated a new set of alliances, confirmed or transformed professional autonomy, and located the risk of birth defects with the recipients of the drug.

Sociologist Ulrich Beck has made the unequal distribution of risk—adverse effects of industrialization such as environmental pollution and radioactive fallout—the hallmark of late modern societies.[12] When standardization is introduced after disaster has already struck and the mechanisms and consequences of insufficient regulation are familiar, the advocates of a standardization system might be tempted to install very restrictive, "tightly coupled" provisions to avoid a repeat.[13] Yet, some actors will require more leeway than others in order to secure their cooperation. The designers' mandate is to define collectively and assess everyone's trustworthiness and dependability and decide who carries the most risk. Physicians, for example, are not waiting for thalidomide manufacturers to redefine their professional jurisdiction in treating patients and prescribing drugs. They are busy defending the boundaries of their own professional autonomy levels with, among others, government regulators, alternative medicine, "web doctors," and managed care. If the proposed thalidomide system fails to consolidate their professional position, they might not sign on. The designers of the standard will need to interest actors in the proposed system, or find a way to force their participation.[14] In the case of thalidomide, the task facing the system designers is to redefine already politically contested autonomy levels of each actor while introducing a toxic substance.

In sum, the standardized distribution system will need to achieve simultaneously three contradictory requirements:

1. *Access:* the distribution system should facilitate access by patients who can benefit from the drug.
2. *Control:* the distribution system should contain safety checks to minimize the risk of fetal exposure, and track any resulting birth defects or neurotoxicity.
3. *Manageability:* the safety checks in the distribution system cannot be too cumbersome because otherwise physicians will be unwilling to prescribe the drug, patients will be unwilling to ask for or take the drug through legitimate channels, and pharmacies will be unwilling

to dispense the drug, resulting in unregulated black market thalidomide.

We explore the normalization of risk to toxic exposure via a standardized distribution system with an outline of the proposed standard, and the reaction of the major actors to the proposal at a public FDA hearing and an NIH meeting. This chapter is largely based on transcripts of two public hearings on thalidomide in 1997, one held by the FDA and the other by the NIH.[15]

THE STANDARDIZED S.T.E.P.S. PROGRAM

Thalidomide was first synthesized in 1954 by Kunz in Germany as an antihistamine, and was introduced as a sedative in 1956 by the German company Chemie Grunenthal. The drug was marketed as a sedative and mild hypnotic under fifty-one brand names in forty-six countries, particularly in Europe, Canada, Australia, South America, and Japan. It quickly became the third largest-selling drug in Europe, because of its prompt action, lack of hangover effect, and apparent safety. In many European countries, thalidomide was available over the counter and physicians prescribed it to pregnant women to combat morning sickness.

In September 1960, the FDA received a new drug application for thalidomide. The application was assigned to a new medical officer, Frances Kelsey, who uncovered serious safety problems with the drug—specifically the possibility of peripheral neuritis, a form of neurotoxicity. Despite repeated pressures from the company and agency superiors, Kelsey delayed approval of the drug and requested additional information from the company. In 1961, while the application was still pending, very serious side effects of the drug were reported in Australia, Germany, and Japan. Johns Hopkins pediatrician Dr. Helen Taussig and journalist Morton Mintz sensitized the U.S. audience to the devastation abroad. As a result of those reports, thalidomide was not approved for marketing in the United States. Yet, the drug manufacturer had already distributed over two and a half million tablets to 1,267 doctors who had prescribed the drug to 19,822 patients, including 3,760 women of childbearing age.[16] As a result ten thalidomide babies were born in the United States.

Worldwide, more than 10,000 babies were born with serious birth defects due to exposure to thalidomide. Most visibly, infants had stunted, flipper-like extremities with missing fingers, and absence of the proximal portion of the limb or absence of entire limbs (phocomelia). Many infants also had affected internal organs. These birth defects were not reproduced in the few early animal models used to evaluate thalidomide (but neither were the sedative properties of the drug). After the thalidomide disaster, studies in which pregnant rabbits were given thalidomide produced the phocomelia birth defects.[17]

Critics and supporters of the FDA agree that the averted thalidomide disaster brought the agency under renewed public scrutiny. Since 1906, the FDA's role was largely limited to checking whether drug labels accurately reflected descriptions of the drug's effects. In 1938, a wave of sulfanilamide deaths had empowered the agency to impose stricter labeling and safety requirements, but it was still the FDA's burden to demonstrate that a drug was not safe in order to keep it off the market. If the agency did not formulate its objections within a fixed time period, a drug automatically became marketable. Once approved, a drug was virtually immune to FDA challenge.

The thalidomide disaster generated momentum for drug regulation among the general public, the Kennedy administration, and legislators, turning the FDA from a modest agency into one of the world's strongest and strictest regulatory bodies.[18] The thalidomide episode was the catalyst of Congress passing the 1962 Kefauver–Harris amendments to the Food, Drug, and Cosmetic Act.[19] These amendments, which had been lingering in congressional committees for years as antitrust legislation, required that drug manufacturers not only had to prove the safety but also the efficacy of the drugs they intended to distribute on the U.S. market. All new drug applications were required to show the drug's safety for use under conditions prescribed in the proposed drug label and were required to show evidence of effectiveness through adequate, well-controlled studies. Finally, the identity, strength, quality, and purity of the drug had to be established through information of quality control, and chemical process used by the manufacturer. Also, the FDA had to take positive action to approve a new drug application before it could be marketed, in contrast with default approval if the FDA did not disapprove the application within six months. These changes not only applied to new drug applications, but to all drugs on the market at the

time. The effects of the amendments were immediate. In the decade before Congress passed the amendments, the FDA approved an average
of 46.2 new single drug entities a year. In the decade after Kefauver–
Harris, the number of approved new single drugs fell to 15.7 a year.[20]
Observers agree that the amendments installed important public health
protections, while at the same time lengthening the drug development
process and skyrocketing the economic cost of drug approval.[21]

It is difficult to exaggerate the symbolic meaning thalidomide had
and still has for the FDA. For decades, the teratogenic effects of thalidomide represented the need for drug regulation and were at the heart
of the FDA's identity. During the advisory committee meeting, Lou
Morris, chief of the division of drug marketing, advertising, and communications at the FDA, summed up thalidomide's importance: "It
does remind us that we have a very important job and that what we
do has huge implications for individual patients and the country as a
whole. . . . [Discussing thalidomide] is symbolic for us because it means
an awful lot about defining who we are and what we do."[22]

After the thalidomide disaster of the 1960s, the compound did not
disappear.[23] Scientists were fascinated by the drug's properties, and
conducted animal research to map the drug's toxicology and pharmacology. Thalidomide continued a thriving underground existence in scientific laboratories, funded by pharmaceutical companies eager to learn
more about its potential while avoiding its devastating powers. In 1965,
an Israeli physician used thalidomide as a sedative for patients with
leprosy (Hansen's disease) and noted that patients who had a tissue
inflammatory syndrome called erythema nodosum leprosum (ENL) responded positively to the drug. Since then, the World Health Organization has recommended thalidomide as the treatment of choice for ENL.
In 1975, the FDA approved thalidomide for leprosy treatment under an
investigational new drug permission (IND) held by the country's major
leprosy treatment center in Carville, Louisiana.

By the 1990s, laboratory research indicated that thalidomide's anti-
inflammatory and immunemodulary agency had potential as a treatment with relatively few side effects for a virtually endless list of immunologic, rheumatologic, hematologic, and oncologic disorders, including AIDS wasting syndrome.[24] Several medical researchers asked
for permission to test and apply thalidomide, prompting the FDA to
form a Thalidomide Working Group in 1994 to develop a uniform in-

formed consent form and a patient information brochure. The next year, the FDA called a meeting of pharmaceutical companies asking them to consider applying for approval to market thalidomide in the United States. The FDA provided two rationales for this strong action. First, the leprosy center in Carville had trouble securing a reliable supplier of thalidomide because no U.S. firm produced the drug. Foreign drug suppliers did not reliably provide the drug, leading to rationing at times and a pharmacologically inconsistent product. The varying quality created a financial burden for the Carville center, and called into question the reliability of the center's clinical research. The second reason was more pressing. Biomedical researchers intended to test thalidomide's effectiveness on conditions such as AIDS wasting syndrome in clinical trials. But the AIDS community did not wait for the trial results: once AIDS activists found out that thalidomide could be used as a treatment for throat and mouth ulcers and to counteract the massive loss of body mass and weight, drug buyer clubs imported the drug from Mexico and Brazil and made it available in the United States via mail-order, sometimes without a name or label on it. Concerned with the illegal distribution of this potentially dangerous drug, the FDA's goal was to make thalidomide legally available while regulating its use.

A small New Jersey company, Celgene, took up the FDA's challenge and submitted a new drug application for the use of thalidomide to treat ENL. Because there are only 100 to 200 new cases of ENL diagnosed in the United States each year, Celgene was able to make the application under the Orphan Drug Act of 1983, which encourages companies to develop drugs for conditions with a low number of patients. As part of the approval system, the company proposed the most stringent drug distribution system in U.S. history, the System for Thalidomide Education and Prescribing Safety (S.T.E.P.S.) program.

Celgene presented scientific data about the safety, efficacy, and indications of thalidomide to the FDA's Dermatologic and Ophthalmic Drugs Advisory Committee meeting in September 1997. The FDA asked the members of that committee to answer eight questions about Celgene's application based on scientific and clinical data, and offer their recommendations to the FDA, which has the final decision and approval power. The committee consisted of nine dermatologists, four ophthalmologists, one biostatistician, and one consumer representative. Because it was a public meeting, any organization could present

an opinion about the drug under consideration: in this case, thalidomide victims, obstetricians, and neurologists were invited to provide
additional information. At the time of the meeting, FDA scientists had
already issued primary and secondary reviews of the company's clinical and toxicological data and a division director had issued a memo
disapproving the application for thalidomide. Yet, the director of the
FDA's office of drug evaluation explained at the beginning of the public advisory meeting that the decision was not set in stone. Working
within a system of supervisory oversight, other directors could write
over-riding memoranda. Because of the important symbolic value of
thalidomide, the FDA staff repeatedly emphasized that the advisory
committee's recommendations would carry a heavy weight in their decision making.

The pivotal question at the meeting was whether thalidomide's benefits outweighed its risks.[25] Among the committee members present at
the meeting, only one member voted no, and another abstained from
the vote. Because the approval of thalidomide had ramifications beyond
ENL, the committee devoted a significant amount of time to discussing
suggestions to improve the company's proposed standardized distribution system.

Based on input from the Thalidomide Victims Association of Canada,[26] neuroscientists, physicians, teratologists, potential patients, academic public health officials, patient advocacy groups, women's health
activists, staff from the CDC, FDA, and NIH, and researchers who implemented a system for a teratogenic acne medication (Accutane) and
an antischizophrenic drug that might cause granular cyrtosis (Clozaril),
Celgene proposed the following state-of-the-art system:[27]

- education of physicians, pharmacists, and patients
- contraceptive counseling by the prescribing physician, or by a referring physician if the prescribing physician does not feel capable, competent, or willing to provide adequate contraceptive counseling
- regimen of pregnancy testing for women with childbearing potential
- informed consent of patients (copies of the forms go to the patient,
  physician, registry, and pharmacy)
- managed distribution
- mandatory outcomes registry survey

At the time of the meetings, Celgene envisioned the following standardized script: when a patient and a physician agree that thalidomide

would be the most appropriate therapy, the physician counsels the patient, using material from Celgene. If the patient understands the risks and responsibilities involved with taking the drug, the patient signs the informed consent form agreeing to participate in a registry survey. The physician then files a copy of the informed consent form, and may write a prescription for no more than four weeks' worth of thalidomide (which cannot be automatically refilled). At that time, male patients receive extra counseling about dangers of pill sharing and are told to use a condom when engaging in sexual activity with a woman of child-bearing age. Female patients receive contraceptive counseling, either by the prescribing physician or through referral to a gynecologist. Before women begin taking the drug, they are required to provide a negative pregnancy test before therapy (or proof of missed periods for twenty-four months, indicating menopause),[28] and delay therapy until simultaneously initiating two forms of effective contraception after their next menstrual period. The patient then goes to a pharmacist who is registered and certified in the S.T.E.P.S. program. Pharmacies can dispense thalidomide for only four weeks at a time. The drug will be packaged in a blister pack with clear warnings, including the photograph of an affected infant. Dispensing can occur only if an informed consent form is presented, and subsequent refills require a new prescription. Each patient will be registered into a tracking system. The survey registry will track compliance with the program on a monthly basis for female patients and on a three-month basis for male patients. Both the FDA and Celgene will monitor the data from the registry, although no specifics were given regarding the frequency of the monitoring or any enforcement actions.

Compared to the average clinical practice guidelines aimed at clinicians, Celgene proposed a standard that would coordinate the actions of diverse groups. Where clinical practice guidelines offer recommendations that give professionals wide leeway, the standardized S.T.E.P.S. program required close compliance to the tasks spelled out in the standard. And while the clinical practice guideline derived much of its authority from a scientific evaluation of evidence, the newness of the drug distribution program led to an unprecedented set of arrangements not backed up with scientific evidence. In comparison to clinical practice guidelines the aims of the standardized S.T.E.P.S. system seem more ambitious and compliance more important to its success. The proposal for the standardized drug distribution program was discussed at the FDA advisory committee meeting, and the members of different groups involved in the program offered their opinions about exactly where the risks and responsibilities lie, how they should be addressed, and which aspects of the proposal should be elaborated or changed. As a link between the drug manufacturer and the patient, the distribution system would confirm or alter power relationships, professional boundaries, agency, and responsibilities of a number of intermediaries. The system not only standardizes the distribution of thalidomide, but also the risk of birth defects with their legal and financial accountability. In the next sections, we address how the major players—physicians, pharmacists, patients, thalidomide victims, the FDA, Celgene, and the drug itself—influenced and redefined this system, how in turn the players' jurisdictions and identities were redefined by the system, and how this process made the risk of fetal exposure acceptable.[29] Our goal is to explore the extent to which members of each group helped to negotiate and stabilize a set of knowledge claims about the management of thalidomide-induced fetal abnormality.

RISK OF FETAL EXPOSURE IN THE S.T.E.P.S. PROGRAM

Physicians

Physicians are the first point of access in the proposed distribution system. They will receive information about the drug and its risks from Celgene, and will be asked to inform their patients about the dangers associated with taking thalidomide. They will also be asked to counsel patients about the use of birth control, in effect, "playing the role of the social worker"[30] in ensuring that women understand the need for contraception, and then ensuring that they are able to get access to it. If a prescribing physician does not feel qualified or comfortable counseling female patients about contraception, Celgene will provide referrals to gynecologists who will do so. After informing their patients about the risks and responsibilities associated with taking thalidomide, physicians have the patients complete informed consent forms, which are filed at the physicians' offices. The physicians then register the patients in the registry system.

But the physician's role is not over once the prescription for thalidomide is written. Patients must return for a new prescription every four weeks, and it is important that the physician monitor all patients carefully for neurotoxicity, and female patients for pregnancy. It was unclear, however, to what extent physicians would be willing or able to perform this unusually high level of monitoring. During the NIH meeting, some participants questioned the likelihood that physicians will follow through with these counseling and monitoring responsibilities. A woman's health advocate stated that some physicians do not adequately counsel their patients about the risks and benefits of treatment and suggested that educational information about off-label use be included in the packet.[31] The Canadian Thalidomide Victims Association representative, Randolph Warren, also noted that "we are not convinced that doctors will give consistent warnings and that doctors are necessarily aware of all aspects of their patients."[32] In turn, physicians questioned the degree to which the current health system would support such a time-intensive counseling system.[33] If the patient is covered by managed care, the physician could run into a number of barriers that may reduce the likelihood of being able to monitor patients according to the S.T.E.P.S. program rules. Managed care companies may set time limits on patient visits;[34] limit drug availability (particularly contraceptives); set caps on treatment costs; or limit second opinions.[35]

Physicians' discretion also poses a challenge to the viability of the distribution system. Although the physician's role is spelled out strongly in the S.T.E.P.S. program, physicians still have considerable flexibility and autonomy when making treatment decisions. Most important, physicians have a professional prerogative to prescribe drugs for indications other than those for which the drug was approved ("off-label" prescribing). Physicians' ability to prescribe off-label erodes the control mechanisms built into the distribution system, because it allows physicians to experiment with the drug. The FDA's consumer advocate, Thalidomiders, discussion participants, a lawyer, and some medical researchers expressed deep concern about off-label use and pressed repeatedly for a restriction of thalidomide. One physician suggested that physicians who prescribed off-label would have to inform their patients that they were engaging in experimental use.[36] According to one of the lawyers who spoke at the meetings, physicians may have the legal prerogative to prescribe off-label, but they do it at their own peril, risking greater legal liability.[37] FDA officials, the drug company, and practicing physicians resisted any off-label restriction on the grounds that physicians' legal professional rights should not be undermined. One physician defended this professional prerogative, stating that "The responsibility for using [thalidomide] wisely falls I think with the medical profession."[38] But as an audience participant noted, precedents for restricting off-label use do exist. Methadone, for example, may only be prescribed for well-defined indications.

Although physicians' full compliance with S.T.E.P.S. program seemed questionable and physicians' prescribing practice constituted a risk for congenital malformations, the only check on physicians' behavior is the administrative paper trail created by the informed consent procedure. Instead, the distribution system gives great latitude to physicians: they make the initial decision about the appropriateness of thalidomide therapy, decide whether the patient is sufficiently informed, follow up with patients if more prescriptions are needed, and maintain the right to prescribe off-label. The system thus preserves and validates physicians' professional and clinical autonomy[39] and does not locate the risk of fetal exposure in the medical profession.

Patients

While consumer and health advocates rather cautiously questioned the willingness of doctors to follow the drug distribution requirements, many of the physicians involved in the advising process—academics, clinicians, public health officials, laboratory researchers—suggested numerous potential complications regarding the patient's part in the distribution system. Patients' opportunities for noncompliance varied, depending on whether the discussion was about patients in general, female patients, or specific patient subpopulations (such as people with AIDS). In the end, however, the drug distribution system relied upon reproductive surveillance, resulting in an erosion of patient autonomy.

Many factors enter into patients' willingness and ability to follow a drug protocol within the context of their everyday lives. During the meetings, physicians who had been involved with prior efforts to change patients' behavior described them as complex actors, with varying degrees of skills and reliability. The physicians pointed out that the potential population of thalidomide patients is very heterogeneous: this fact calls into question the feasibility of truly standardizing behavior across patients in the distribution system. Potential patients would have varying levels of literacy (with 20 percent of the population considered illiterate and another 20 percent functionally illiterate);[40] existing knowledge about the drug;[41] formal education, income, and insurance;[42] knowledge of English due to recent immigration status;[43] sickness;[44] and varying levels of contraceptive skills.[45] They would also come with varying beliefs about sexual intercourse, contraception, and abortion. In addition, some patients could be expected to do their own research on available treatments and then actively seek them out; these patients might want a greater voice in deciding which treatment they will receive.

Perception of risk may vary tremendously among the potential patient population. Over 50 percent of people over the age of 45 have very vivid associations with the word *thalidomide.* But only about one-third of people under the age of 45 (largely the reproductive age) know of the drug's history.[46] But it is not enough for patients to know that there is a risk. They must also understand how to prevent that risk from becoming a reality in their own lives. That kind of behavioral change requires that patients believe that the risk is real, intend to perform the change, and have the skills and environmental resources to make the change effectively. According to a discussion during the meetings, the most important environmental resource is the availability of contraceptives. If patients are not easily able to get access to contraceptives, because of lack of insurance or money or other barriers,[47] the entire system may be compromised.

Three patient populations received special attention during the FDA and NIH meetings: leprosy patients, HIV and AIDS patients, and female patients. Leprosy patients had been receiving thalidomide for decades and were, at least on paper, the intended drug recipients. Fueled by biblical associations with impurity, the leprosy population in the United States has had a long and sad history of civil rights violations as a consequence of mandatory institutionalization.[48] The Carville leprosy center required surgical sterilization or proof of menopause for female outpatients, and required that female inpatients receive two forms of contraception and weekly pregnancy tests.[49] In the public meetings, the Carville experience with leprosy patients was interpreted to mean that the risk of thalidomide could be minimized with proper monitoring. No former or current leprosy patients were present to affirm or challenge this portrayal at the meetings.

HIV and AIDS patients, the second patient population discussed at length, offered a bigger challenge for the designers of the distribution system. In contrast with the assumed docility of the leprosy population, people with HIV symbolized demanding, assertive, well-organized, activist-patient bodies. Patient activists from the AIDS epidemic[50] have been aggressive about pressuring doctors for new treatments, or seeking drugs from buyers' clubs if physicians will not dispense them.[51] HIV and AIDS patients, and their activists, therefore represented the real possibility of future thalidomide patients bypassing the regulated distribution system if its requirements were too stringent.

Expected to be the largest consumers of thalidomide, HIV patients may already be participating in demanding therapies, involving as many as twenty-eight pills each day. And some people with AIDS may be living on the socioeconomic fringe, with a significant amount of chaos involved in their lives.[52] Thalidomide may add to that chaos for some patients, on top of figuring out where their next meal will come from, where their next ride to and from the doctor's will come from, whether they will still live in their house, and, for parents, how they will take care of their children. Poor populations may need extra support. Adding to these challenges, some patients may be illicit drug users, and such users do not have a good track record of contraceptive use.[53] An additional problem is posed by the effects of thalidomide itself: it is a sedative, and may impair the judgment of patients who take it,[54] reducing compliance with a contraceptive program.

Female patients were the third key patient population that was discussed during the meetings. Ultimately, the S.T.E.P.S. program aimed to influence their reproductive behavior. During the FDA meetings, women had a limited voice, but their possible future behavior within the distribution system was the subject of heated debate on several occasions. According to the discussion, much of the credit for the success or failure of the S.T.E.P.S. program will fall on female patients' shoulders. Some of the actors during the FDA and NIH meetings trusted women with that responsibility, while others portrayed future female patients as unreliable. Throughout the meetings, women were alternatively described as intelligent decision makers, unsuitable patients, people with varying degrees of ability and reliability, and unruly physical bodies.

Cynthia Pearson, a representative from the National Women's Health Network (NWHN), described women patients as intelligent decision makers, who would make good choices if they understood the risks associated with their behavior. Hers was the one voice that specifically spoke on behalf of future women patients during the FDA and NIH meetings. Pearson advocated that women make their own choices about contraception, rather than having physicians or the FDA make those decisions, and challenged a stereotypical view that "all women who ovulate and have open fallopian tubes are at risk of pregnancy."[55] She emphasized that most women would not want to have babies with birth defects, and would take decisions accordingly after they are informed about the risks associated with taking thalidomide.

The most conservative view of women, as unsuitable patients, was held by some of the research scientists who had been working with thalidomide at the Carville leprosy center. They were accustomed to a clinical situation where zero risk was tolerated and institutionalization was a routine intervention. Leo Yoder, one of the physicians at Carville, advocated that women be required to use two methods of contraception, and stated that ideally, women would use a method "that does not apply to compliance."[56] Others suggested that women should not receive the drug at all, or only making it available to infertile women in clinical trials.

Female patients' bodies were also characterized as varying in ways that the distribution system, and the women themselves, cannot control. By instituting monthly pregnancy tests, the system hopes to guarantee that a pregnant woman will not receive thalidomide. But women often do not have twenty-eight-day cycles,[57] making it unclear at what point in her cycle a woman is being tested, if she is tested every twenty-eight days. Technological issues compound this problem: it takes nine to ten days for a serum pregnancy test to become positive, so a negative test only shows that the woman is not ten days or more pregnant. But the sensitive period is twenty-one to thirty-six days.[58] To be absolutely sure that a pregnant woman does not take the drug, women would have to be tested every ten days. The FDA did not require this frequency of testing, because it feared that the requirement would be too stringent and drive people to the buyers' clubs.[59]

In the end, a discursive construction of women as unreliable and unpredictable overwhelmingly shaped the S.T.E.P.S. program. In contrast to the relatively few controlling provisions for physicians, women's knowledge and behavior is counseled, questioned, verified, checked, tested, rechecked, and then continuously monitored via a compliance survey. Largely based upon the accumulated knowledge of AIDS prevention research,[60] the final version of the S.T.E.P.S. program is aimed at modifying female sexual behavior. If a woman has not undergone a hysterectomy or been sterilized, or has menstruated in the twenty-four months preceding thalidomide treatment, she must agree to two forms of contraception. One of those methods must be highly effective (e.g., IUD, hormonal, tubal ligation, or partner's vasectomy), and be used in combination with one effective method (e.g., condom, diaphragm, or cervical cap). Women must also produce a written negative pregnancy test that was conducted no more than twenty-four hours prior to beginning treatment with THALOMID™. After receiving the drug, women of childbearing potential must receive a pregnancy test every week for the first four weeks, then every four weeks thereafter if their menstrual cycles are regular. If her cycle is irregular, a woman must receive a pregnancy test every two weeks thereafter. If all else fails, emergency contraception will be made available to female patients.

All patients, regardless of their sex, are monitored to some extent within the proposed S.T.E.P.S. program. Patients are instructed that they should not donate blood. Female patients cannot breast feed while on THALOMID™, and male patients are instructed to use a condom every time that they have sexual intercourse with a woman (even if they have undergone a vasectomy) and are not allowed to donate sperm.[61] Each patient must fill out informed consent forms, take a quiz, register via a survey enrollment form, and participate in the registry survey (monthly for female patients and quarterly for male patients). This confidential survey asks questions about sexual behavior, pill sharing, and use of contraception, and requests the results of pregnancy tests. Every patient is assumed to be able and willing to freely discuss his or her sexual behavior with physicians and survey researchers.

Susan Cohen, the official consumer advocate on the FDA panel, asked repeatedly whether abortion would be made available to a woman who preferred not to carry an affected child, and what measures would be taken for people who did not believe in abortion. The original thalidomide disaster in the 1960s strengthened the argument for the legalization of abortion when the media reported the case of a middle-class woman who had to travel abroad to abort a thalidomide fetus. The FDA transcripts offer an interesting ethnomethodological moment when the word *abortion* was mentioned. A reader can sense the desperate scrambling to answer other parts of the consumer advocate's question and avoid the topic. During the meetings, the FDA and Celgene never addressed the abortion question. The final S.T.E.P.S. package also does not contain information about abortion as a health care option, but instead warns that "THALOMID™ does not induce abortion of the fetus and should never be used for contraception."[62]

The invasive and elaborate measures to assure patient compliance show that the system designers saw the real risk of fetal exposure as residing with patients, particularly female patients, rather than the professional actors within the system. Although an ethicist at the NIH meeting quoted an attorney stating that "a woman has no legal or moral duty to be a procreative saint,"[63] the system singles out female patients. It is also clear that the system focuses on sexual activity and pregnancy as the locus of risk, not fetal exposure, even though a Celgene representative claimed that the opposite was true.[64] The standardized distribution system assumes that a woman is in charge of contraception, reproductive decisions, and her sexual relationships. But at the same time, all women wishing to take THALOMID™ are also presumed to be heterosexually active unless they can prove hysterectomy or menopause. Women's sexual behavior and their bodies are ultimately untrustworthy. At every point where female patients' behavior was interpreted, the strictest control (short of institutionalization) was chosen. The system works from the assumption that women are willing to trade a close supervision and regulation of their sexuality and reproductive privacy for access to a potentially life-saving drug.[65] Women are not trusted to make decisions to protect their unborn children.[66]

Thalidomiders

Randolph Warren, the CEO of the Thalidomide Victims Association of Canada, played a crucial role in developing the S.T.E.P.S. program. Warren attended the FDA and NIH advisory committee meetings, speaking for the handful of U.S. thalidomide victims, the thalidomide victims and mothers in Canada, and future thalidomide babies. During those meetings, he consistently and vocally demanded that the program do its best to minimize the risk of thalidomide babies being born in the United States. Prior to the FDA meetings, Warren worked closely with Celgene to develop the S.T.E.P.S. program. Although he was unhappy[67] about thalidomide being available in the United States, he preferred FDA regulation of the drug to the current situation, stating that "It pains us, but we have come to this conclusion, that we're forced to prefer the regulation of thalidomide because we are so much more afraid of thalidomide being available as it is today or having it relegated to a secret world controlled by so few doctors and scientists, who we won't disrespect, but we would rather see it be a very public controlled environment."[68]

Warren saw his role as an educator. He and the other members of his organization understood the potential impact of the drug in a way that none of the other actors could, and they wanted to serve as a lighthouse, showing the danger that lay ahead. It was important to Warren that the dangers be stated clearly, using photographs of infants and videos of adult thalidomide victims, to show the extent of the damage that thalidomide could cause. He believed that education was the key to protecting future babies: if women could see the devastating damage that thalidomide could cause, they would prevent it. Throughout the meetings, he asked, "What will you tell the thalidomide baby that inevitably will be born?" and demanded that Celgene work to develop nonteratogenic substitutes for thalidomide, eliminating the need for the drug in the future. Warren did not sidestep the abortion question: he stated that although abortion is each woman's choice, it could not be considered a safety net. Every abortion would be another death as a result of thalidomide and his organization aimed for zero fetal exposure. In addition, "people should not be forced to sign anything that would force them to have an abortion should a thalidomider be born because we have some quality of life and some right to be here."[69]

As the living embodiment of the drug's major risk,[70] the Thalidomiders had some direct effects on the S.T.E.P.S. program. They critiqued the drug packaging, offered to participate in the creation of an informative video to educate future patients, and proposed to make themselves available as counselors for future thalidomide babies. The final educational package includes a letter from the Canadian Thalidomide Victims Association, which is addressed to prospective patients and physicians. A picture of a smiling thalidomide baby is included in the information folder. In turn, the renewed attention to thalidomide and the S.T.E.P.S. program gave the Thalidomiders a forum in which to validate their concerns and questions. Aware of their living symbolic value and their dwindling numbers, Thalidomiders presented themselves as the spokespeople of the future affected children. The Thalidomiders advocated for a zero tolerance of the risk of fetal exposure, wanting to prevent the birth of similarly affected babies in the future, even if that meant that a picture of a Thalidomider would be used as a deterrent. Their main goal was to prevent more babies from being affected. Warren sadly expressed the irony that Thalidomiders "cannot fight thalidomide. It wins every time."[71]

Pharmacists

In the proposed thalidomide distribution system, pharmacists are required to submit to external control, but make important professional gains. Pharmacies must participate in a registry program in order to be able to order thalidomide from the wholesaler. Pharmacies will also be required to enter information about the prescription into an on-line system, which will verify that the patient is registered, and then authorize the pharmacy to distribute the drug. Bruce Williams, the Celgene architect of the distribution system, explained this final step was designed to monitor pharmacists' compliance: "a portion of a database will be carved out to actually have the pharmacist tracking and recording information on this patient so that we'd be in a position to monitor that the pharmacist was in fact complying with the program."[72] Yet, pharmacists play a key role as the last link in the distribution chain. This gatekeeper role changes pharmacists' professional jurisdiction: pharmacists are expected to ensure that the patient is registered and that he or she has read and signed the informed consent form, and determine that the physician wrote the prescription correctly (for only twenty-eight days, with no refills). If any of those conditions are not met, the pharmacist has the authority not to dispense the drugs and to send the patient back to the physician.[73]

These new requirements redefine the traditional boundaries between physicians and pharmacists, asking pharmacists to take a much larger role in distributing the drug than is typical. Pharmacists check on physicians' prescribing behavior and verify whether the physician correctly explained the implications of participating in the drug program. The distribution extends pharmacists' usual role in interacting with patients, which is to fill the prescription, and answer any questions that the patients may have about the drug. Since the 1970s, pharmacists' work has become increasingly routinized, and they now spend much of their time performing the administrative and clerical tasks associated with filling prescriptions and obtaining insurance information.[74] Within this context, the S.T.E.P.S. program gives pharmacists power and discretion in distributing thalidomide.[75]

The pharmacists at the NIH meeting welcomed this increased role. A spokesperson stated that pharmacists "oral counseling" of patients is becoming a standard of practice.[76] A representative of the American Pharmaceutical Association argued for acknowledgment that pharmacists are already active in patient education and noted that they are lobbying to reflect such change in pharmacy practice acts at state level.[77] In addition, the pharmacists also suggested that the drug companies should compensate them for their increased responsibilities.[78] Other participants in the discussion, mostly physicians, saw problems in an changed role for pharmacists. They pointed to the rapid turnover and rotation of staff in many pharmacies, creating the possibility that the pharmacist dispensing thalidomide was not trained to do so, and suggested limiting the number of pharmacies distributing thalidomide to six or seven centers in the country. They also worried about mail-in pharmacies. Furthermore, some meeting participants were concerned about how pharmacists would handle increased liability under the S.T.E.P.S. program. According to a lawyer at the NIH meeting, case law traditionally has protected pharmacies from liability: "when push comes to shove within the legal system, they hide behind this facade of case law that really insulates them from any type of professional responsibility for the harm that they cause."[79]

Just as the physicians' professional and clinical autonomy was not seriously questioned, little action was taken regarding these concerns about pharmacists' willingness and ability to follow the S.T.E.P.S. guidelines. The final version of the distribution system does not add extra safeguards to increase pharmacists' compliance. Instead, the pharmacists' role in the system expands their professional jurisdiction to include gatekeeping functions.

FDA

Thalidomide has tremendous symbolic value in the history of the FDA. The agency's regulatory powers were strengthened in 1961 by its reluctance to approve the drug. The social-political context in which the FDA makes decisions about drug approval applications, however, has changed significantly in the almost forty years since the thalidomide tragedy. The FDA is working in a macro-political climate of less regulation, less bureaucracy, and more independent decision making by consumers.[80] Currently, there are calls for expanded access to clinical trials (notably by women and minorities), pressure from the pharmaceutical industry to accelerate approval for drug distribution and marketing, a strengthened antiabortion movement, treatment activism (especially by HIV/AIDS activists), and stronger consumer awareness. Often, patients are now more involved in their treatment than they were in the past, and look to the FDA to provide them with a statement of the risks associated with drugs, so that they can participate in managing that risk.[81] The FDA's role is still to monitor the safety of drugs, but the agency is strongly criticized if it is seen as getting in the way of distributing promising new therapies to people with severe diseases.[82]

When it invited drug companies to rethink thalidomide, the FDA created a more proactive role for itself as a federal consumer protection agency that regulates industry based on scientific data.[83] But the invitation to apply, the less rigorous application process under the orphan drug status,[84] and the disregard for the agency's own safety experts who argued that the application did not meet scientific criteria,[85] created the impression that the approval of thalidomide was virtually guaranteed. Indeed, Warren noted, "To be critical, as far as I'm concerned, the first application should have been an honest application that was involving HIV/AIDS wasting."[86]

Although the FDA played a key role in paving the way for the distribution of thalidomide, and in the development of the S.T.E.P.S. program, it will play a backstage role in the implementation of the system. In response to a question during the NIH meeting about who will be responsible for overseeing the distribution system when it is in action, one FDA representative stated that "I think it's the responsibility of all of us. That's one reason the organizers put together this meeting, because every group represented here, from the patient groups, to academia, to government research, to government regulation, to consumer groups, to lawyers, and to companies doing drug development, all are going to have to contribute if we're going to make it go forward correctly, I think. It can't just be the responsibility of one group."[87] From a consumer's point of view, the distribution system would have had extra teeth if the FDA had insisted on a clearly defined set of criteria to evaluate the adverse effects of THALOMID™. A lawyer who represents injured victims asked the haunting rhetorical question: "Just how many children will need to be harmed by this drug before the risks of the drug are deemed to outweigh the benefits?"[88] He added that in his home state of Michigan, once the FDA has approved a drug, it is deemed to be safe. No lawsuit can be brought unless it can be demonstrated that the FDA approval had been procured by fraud. Although the FDA has a voluntary postmarketing reporting system—a database consisting of adverse drug reactions—in place, it remained unclear at what point the agency might step in to further restrict access to the drug. Researchers estimate that only about 5 to 10 percent of adverse reactions are reported and that causality is difficult to establish.[89]

Some observers have noted the FDA's deft political move in the thalidomide case:[90] the FDA showed its sensitivity to the needs of patients, while taking responsibility for the outcomes of a minute number of leprosy cases and avoiding responsibility for the estimated thousands of off-label prescriptions. Although this is not such a watershed event, compared with the first time the FDA came in contact with thalidomide, its approval of thalidomide reflects the course the FDA hopes to set in the future as a regulatory agency. The FDA sent the message to its critics that within the current regulatory system, it is possible to approve even thalidomide. Major reform, budget cuts, or loosening of restrictions are not warranted. Once again, the FDA managed to transform itself in interaction with thalidomide.

Celgene

Celgene took primary responsibility for developing the S.T.E.P.S. program, but sought the advice of many different groups during that process. Even before the company presented the program in the public FDA and NIH meetings, representatives had consulted with thalidomide victims, physicians, future patients, the FDA,[91] and other potential actors in the system. They also worked closely with the staff at the Slone Epidemiology Unit at Boston University, which had previously operated a pregnancy prevention program for a teratogenic acne medication called Accutane. That program apparently had high, but by no means perfect, levels of compliance.

Most participants in the discussion complimented Celgene for designing such a well-thought-out system. The strategic negotiations with multiple social worlds (notably the Thalidomide Victims Association) showed that the company had taken a lot of responsibility for informing patients, physicians, and pharmacists, and for tracking compliance in the design of the system. But in the end the program works through delegation, largely independently from Celgene. Once the system is put in place, the company's role is limited to distributing drugs after informed consent is documented. It is left up to physicians, patients, and pharmacists to ensure that the system is kept on track. Celgene will receive data from the Slone registry, but it remains unclear how these data will be evaluated and with what consequences. Although the company showed an impressive sensitivity in designing the system in order to secure FDA approval, their initiatives could be interpreted as largely legally defensive in case a thalidomide baby is born. It is important to note that the Accutane pregnancy prevention system has already withstood several legal challenges. One of the causes for public outrage in the original thalidomide disaster was the difficulty victims had in locating liability and winning compensation from the manufacturer and the distributors.[92] Celgene distributed the benefit of the scientific doubt according to its legal interests.[93]

The major change for Celgene with the design and approval of the S.T.E.P.S. program is that the company made the coveted transition from a research company to a drug manufacturer. FDA approval puts Celgene in a strong position to furnish thalidomide to many patient populations. With the FDA's approval of THALOMID™, Celgene's stock initially rose, and the company recently has added new divisions. Such growth has its own financial risks, but those are existentially different from the risk of potential future thalidomide victims.

Thalidomide

Thalidomide has been reevaluated and redeemed. Once, it was an over-the-counter remedy for insomnia and morning sickness that caused devastating birth defects among infants. Now, it is an "essential" drug for patients with painful and often life-threatening diseases who are otherwise untreatable, such as people with ENL and AIDS wasting syndrome. Thalidomide is allowed to act again in the United States. Because of its "pharmacotherapeutic rehabilitation,"[94] several patient groups have a new outlook on life, physicians have a new tool, pharmacists gain a new opportunity for jurisdictional expansion, the FDA has a new standard for drug distribution, and Celgene has prospects for profit. The rehabilitated thalidomide is the linchpin that holds all those groups together in a new configuration. Thalidomide shapes the individual lives and professional careers of these groups and, in turn, will be defined by the degree to which these groups conform to the S.T.E.P.S. requirements.

To indicate the break with the past, Celgene proposed the name Synovir for the transformed thalidomide. But the discussion participants agreed that Synovir sounded too much like the name of an ordinary antiviral drug, and, to play on the name recognition among people over 45, the name became THALOMID™, with "thalidomide" in brackets. Thalidomide's transformation affected even its visual presentation. Instead of distributing the drug in a bottle, the meeting participants preferred blister packaging with an expiration date.

In constructing the drug distribution system, medical researchers compiled and evaluated the available knowledge about the drug's absorption time, biological equivalency, etiology, toxicity, drug interactions (particularly with oral contraceptives), teratogenicity, peripheral neuropathy, efficiency for ENL, and immunological agency. A comparison with other teratogenic drugs already on the market further drew out the characteristics of thalidomide until a picture of its pharmacological consistency appeared. Instead of a horror drug of the past, thalidomide appeared through the scientific work as any other chemical compound with known toxicological parameters, and, as was stated repeatedly, this picture proved less alarming than some other drugs currently approved by the FDA and widely available by prescription (e.g., Accutane). The discussants chiseled away at thalidomide's symbolic value even further when they emphasized the limitless therapeutic applications of the drug. The result of these defining acts was a symbolic, functional, and therapeutic makeover of thalidomide, and the establishment of a new identity: THALOMID™.

But the drug's identity picture was not complete. Some features remained unknown or controversial. One of the biggest gaps in the drug knowledge was thalidomide's mechanism of action, both generally and in specific conditions. Several hypotheses were circulated of how thalidomide might cause congenital birth defects and neuropathy, but no consensus existed. A number of audience members, including Iris Long from ACT UP/New York,[95] demanded an acknowledgment of the drug's unpredictability in the informed consent form. Other very basic pharmacological data (for example, about dosing) was missing as well, and several participants called for more animal models, clinical trials, and research applications. Some of those new applications might lead to discovering thalidomide's therapeutic role for life-altering conditions instead of life threatening conditions, raising issues about the standard of the drug's risk and benefits. Researchers generally considered the lack of knowledge a stimulus for more research and they expressed cautious excitement about the future of thalidomide. In the final version of the S.T.E.P.S. informed consent form, no disclaimers or warnings about the drug's unknowns were mentioned. A lawyer noted that the lack of clear causal path might limit the legal accountability of people suffering from the adverse effects of the drug, because some congenital malformations occur "naturally" in the general population.

At the same time that the drug distribution system rehabilitated thalidomide, it also put the drug under strict control and severely limited its access to human bodies. Thalidomide is the most regulated drug in U.S. history.[96] The rehabilitation of thalidomide might also carry the seeds of its demise. Because of the enormous therapeutic promise and profit margin, the race is on for an analog with thalidomide's healing qualities but without its teratogenic effects. A Celgene representative referred to the analog as "the holy grail of drug development."[97]

STANDARDIZATION AND THE NORMALIZATION OF RISK

Bolstered by the positive recommendations of the public hearing, in July 1998 the FDA approved Celgene's application to market THALOMID™ in the United States for use in treating ENL. Physicians interested in prescribing THALOMID™ received a folder explaining the different aspects of the S.T.E.P.S. program. The folder contained detailed, standardized guidelines on how to prescribe the drug for female and male patients. Although physicians were required to conduct most of the coordinating work, the drug distribution program ultimately was aimed at surveillance of female patients.

Once a standardized drug distribution system is put in place and seamlessly becomes part of medical practice, it is difficult to have a good overview of the roles of all the different players, and almost impossible to understand the assumptions behind specific guidelines and protocols. Like blocks of computer language copied repeatedly in the public domain and taken for granted, standards slide to the background and become "invisible."[98] The public meetings and debates surrounding the creation of standards offer a rare reflexive space where we can observe the stance the developers took on the "tastes, competencies, motives, aspirations, and political prejudices"[99] of every actor and where they decided to locate risk and responsibility. In this sense, as Leigh Star and Geof Bowker point out, "each standard and each category valorizes some point of view and silences another."[100] In the standardized thalidomide distribution system, silencing and valorizing are inevitably tied to the risk of fetal exposure.

Haunted by the thalidomide disaster, in 1962 Congress gave the FDA unprecedented powers to regulate drugs. In 1998, the same compound with the same teratogenic potential was approved for distribution in the United States. Among the factors that helped to overcome the heavy symbolic legacy of thalidomide and made its distribution possible were the proactive role of the FDA, an evaluation of scientific expertise,[101] cooperation with Thalidomiders, a presentation of the limitless benefits for hard-hit patient populations, the threat of unregulated black-market thalidomide, and the strategically positioned S.T.E.P.S. program. In this chapter, we have highlighted the role of the distribution program in normalizing the risk of congenital malformation.

One of the merits of the standardized S.T.E.P.S. program is that it satisfies the most powerful actors whose collaboration was needed for the system to operate. The designers preserved and enhanced their professional autonomy. Physicians' off-label prescription prerogatives were left untouched, and pharmacists were given desired counseling responsibilities. The federal regulators were satisfied that the proposed drug system set a new precedent for restricted distribution. The fact that thalidomide was approved showed that the current drug regulation system worked and that the agency paid attention to the needs of the pharmaceutical industry and patient populations. The program simultaneously positioned Celgene at the beginning of the distribution chain and minimized the company's participation once the system was put into place. The reluctant Thalidomiders played an important role in educating Celgene and the other actors about thalidomide's dangers. As for the most silent actors, the patients, the system assumes that access to a life-saving drug will be a sufficient incentive to make the program a success. Their submission is subsumed as part of an implied quid pro quo.[102]

The distribution system also clearly identifies women's sexual behavior as the primary locus of risk of congenital malformations. The standardization effort provided a sense of security because it imposed an ideal situation in which fetal exposure should not occur if all actors played their roles. Throughout the debates a consensus emerges that the risk for congenital malformations resides in a distribution of responsibilities. The formalized distribution chain minimized the risk of adverse effects by defining a number of loopholes and then suggesting means to close them off. The risk of a thalidomide baby is defined as the risk of a woman patient taking thalidomide. It bears repeating that controlling women's reproductive behavior is not necessarily the only or most obvious choice: physicians' off-label use or pill sharing among male and female patients could have been the target of control. Or instead of increasing the surveillance of female sexuality, the different actors could have pointed to the availability of abortion as a legal health care choice. By marking women's reproductive behavior as the most important safety valve, the designers perpetuated a distorted view of women as untrustworthy decision makers and delegated control to physicians and pharmacists.

In this case, standardization thus strengthens social inequalities and professional power relationships, revealing assumptions about trust, responsibility, and risk. The result is a new script, a drama in this case, which specifies roles, danger, motivations, and objects of desire. Whether the guidelines of the script will actually be followed remains to be seen. Even in the design phase, the actors recognized the potential to bypass the system (for example, with Mexican thalidomide). As we have shown, a reshuffling of control and leeway—often unanticipated by standard designers—is *necessary* for any standard to function. The careful balance between control, flexibility, and manageability will need to be achieved anew during drug prescription and dispensing. The participants in the debate were aware of the tension between designing and implementing a distribution system, because they stated repeatedly that it was inevitable that thalidomide babies would be born in the United States. One of the lawyers at the meetings worried more specifically that "The impact of noncompliance by literally everyone in the distribution chain is a high likelihood, not an isolated instance."[103] The

lawyer's deeply felt concern stood out because most meeting participants considered the probability of noncompliance insufficient to stop
the distribution of thalidomide. An FDA official stated at the end of the
meetings that enforcing the system "is the responsibility of all of us."[104]
The standardization attempt seemed to have absorbed individual responsibilities and located an ambiguous collective and formalistic responsibility in the distribution system.[105] A physician from the Centers
for Disease Control and Prevention described the S.T.E.P.S. program as
being similar to error prevention analysis systems for medical errors—
"a way of not thinking about individuals, but thinking about a systems
approach to prevent errors—is a nice way to think about it."[106] At the
outset of thalidomide distribution, it seems that the standardized system itself will be to blame, put to trial, and patched up or overhauled
for any adverse effects and not one of the social worlds. The responsibility for adverse effects rests with the distribution chain made up of
interconnecting links.

Similar to Diane Vaughan's analysis of the *Challenger* launch decision,
the end result of the public meetings and the FDA approval process was
the collapse of previously considered deviating results into a new criterion of acceptable risk. The standardized S.T.E.P.S. program leads to a
normalization of risk of birth defects.[107] The FDA and Celgene admitted
up front that the S.T.E.P.S. program would not completely prevent congenital malformations due to thalidomide, yet the standardized distribution system made the residual risk of congenital disability acceptable.
It shifted the cost-benefit ratio in favor of the benefits, by promising to
reduce and control the risk of fetal exposure and disability. While this
normalization of risk might be doable for the current actors in the distribution chain, the question still remains whether this justification of
risk will satisfy the thalidomide babies who will be born.[108]

Epilogue
The Quest for Quality

IN 2000 AND 2001, the U.S. Institute of Medicine published two reports that set a new tone in the ongoing calls for health care reform. In the first report, "To Err is Human: Building a Safer Health System," the Committee on Quality of Health Care in America claimed that medical errors (such as administering wrong drugs, or failing to execute a planned intervention) are a leading cause of death in the United States.[1] Much critique was raised against the precise figures listed and the exact definitions of error.[2] Yet the overall argument of the report—that the U.S. health care environment was not the safe environment that one would expect it to be—was not substantially contested. One year later, the same committee published "Crossing the Quality Chasm: A New Health System for the 21st Century," in which the insights of the first report were generalized to the claim that the overall quality of U.S. health care services was far below standard. Given the amount of resources spent and the motivation of the average health care professional, the committee argued, there is a huge chasm between what the overall quality delivered by the system should be and what it actually is. The committee discerned six dimensions of quality:

1. *Safety* ("patients should not be harmed by the care that is intended to help them")
2. *Effectiveness* (the care given should be evidence-based, and optimally directed at the individual's medical needs)
3. *Patient-centered* (care should respect patients' values, preferences, and expressed needs; services should be organized and integrated around the patients' experience, to maximize physical and emotional comfort; information, communication, and education should be central)

4. *Timeliness* (waiting times and delays before and during care delivery should be minimized; "any high-quality process should flow smoothly")
5. *Efficiency* (care should be directed at getting "the best value for the money spent"; waste through inefficient processes or the execution of noneffective interventions should be reduced)
6. *Equity* (health care should be universally accessible, and the quality of care received should not depend on individuals' personal characteristics such as "gender, race, age, ethnicity, income, education, disability, sexual orientation, or location of residence")[3]

In an unusually critical tone, the committee charges that the current U.S. health care system fails miserably on all these levels. It is highly fragmented, "a nightmare to navigate," "bewildering," and "wasteful." Any journey through it includes many "steps and handoffs that slow down the care process and decrease rather than improve safety." All in all, "our attempts to deliver today's technologies with today's medical production capabilities are the medical equivalent of manufacturing microprocessors in a vacuum tube factory."[4]

This already rather damning conclusion is further aggravated by the fact that the demands on the health care system will increase substantially over the next years. Technological and scientific developments in fields such as genomics will not slow down, the committee argues, and this will significantly add to the complexity of health care delivery. In addition, the incidence of chronic conditions increases rapidly with the rise in life expectancy and medicine's increasing ability to control diseases even if it cannot cure them.

> Meeting this challenge demands a readiness to think in radically new ways about how to deliver health care services and how to assess and improve their quality. Our present efforts resemble a team of engineers trying to break the sound barrier by tinkering with a Model T Ford.[5]

It is generally acknowledged by quality advocates that the committee's overall insights are applicable to most Western countries. The issue of equity might be less significant for countries where lack of health insurance is not such a major issue as it is in the United States. On the other hand, when increasing numbers of patients pay high fees to private clinics to bypass waiting lists in the United Kingdom or the Netherlands, equity is at stake there as well.

What are the solutions that the committee brings to the fore? Much of its recommendations restate the need for evidence-based guidelines and information technology that we have discussed in this book. The report stresses the importance of setting clear performance standards for health care services. These should span all dimensions of quality, addressing, for example, minimal levels of timeliness, patient information, achieved health benefits, and so forth. Several indicators or performance measures should be developed for each dimension, for each disease category, and for each type of care delivered. An integrated diabetes care service, for example, could be scored on the percentage of preventable complications of diabetes, or the adequacy of hemoglobin A1c control.[6]

To reach these performance standards, procedural standards such as evidence-based guidelines are a crucial means. When well-designed, adherence to such standards should yield the desired performance standards. When practicing state-of-the-art medicine, after all, the clinical outcomes should be optimal. Similarly, when guidelines encompass how to optimally organize care, following these guidelines should also ensure the patient satisfaction and timeliness achieved in these "best practices." For all of this, terminological and design standards are a sine qua non. Without proper coding of data, for example, it becomes all but impossible to compare performance measurements between institutions. Proper reporting habits and the increased use of information technology should increase the transparency of medical work, and, concurrently, the interoperability between different care providers in the chain of care. The electronic medical record is the core vehicle required to achieve these aims. The IT interoperability necessary for all these information flows, the committee argues, demands the agreement upon many design standards including data encryption, accessibility regulations, forms, and so forth.

More of the Same?

Is there anything new here? Is this evidence-based medicine redux? The emphasis on standardization is a clear continuation of already existing drives, and the calls for transparency, guidelines, the electronic medical record, and so forth sound very familiar. The calls for increased effectiveness, efficiency, equity, timeliness, and patient-centeredness are also hardly new. These same needs were stressed when the first national consensus meetings yielded their first guidelines in the late 1970s and early 1980s. Similarly, these same aims were stressed to promote the coming of the electronic patient record in the United States and Europe during the 1990s.

Safety, and the errors that the 2000 report emphasized, on the other hand, have not been in the forefront recently. Yet related issues were high on the agenda of the American College of Surgeons almost a century ago. In fact, as we mentioned in the introduction, the industrial standardization efforts that fueled the early hospital standardization movement were themselves driven partly by a preoccupation with safety. Just as the American railroads wanted to prevent boilers from exploding and trains from derailing, American hospitals should be safeguarded from surgical errors and equipment failures.

Is there then nothing new under the sun? In her critique of medicine's current obsession with accountability, Carolyn Wiener argues that this focus on quality improvement and performance measures is but an intensification of the earlier standardization efforts. Today's accountability movement, she argues, is unique in its relentless effort to prove to the outside world that resources are spent wisely, and that quality (in all its dimensions) is high and ever-improving. Publishing mortality rates of individual surgeons on the Internet and making "report cards" with which patients and insurers can assess the quality of health care providers are new developments. Yet in her view, this quest for accountability directly emerged from the rationalization attempts dating from the 1970s and 1980s and farther back: the construction of guidelines, hospital accreditation efforts, the increased calls for transparency, and so forth.[7]

To argue that this quest must remain elusive, then, Wiener can draw upon the old arguments brought to bear against these earlier rationalization efforts as well. Contemporary health care is simply too complex for any such comprehensive standardization attempt to succeed. Drawing upon the seminal work of Anselm Strauss and co-authors (including herself), she argues that the care process "cannot be fully standardized." The speed of technical developments, the appetite of people for more and better health care, and the organizational complexity of the health care system are "the dynamics that contribute to the complexity of medical care, that vary the work of caring for patients, that cause coordination problems, that defy simple solutions, and that confound the notion of outcome measures and treatment based on algorithms."[8] More evidence will never change this. All in all, she argues, "there is no such thing as a standard illness or standard patient."[9] More standardization simply means less life in the health care system and dehumanization of care. Ultimately, depleted of its vital juices—the practical, nonstandardizable situated work of health care workers—all health care processes will grind to a halt.

We feel that such criticism has largely outlived its usefulness. Of course, as a counterforce against the never-ending hype of "more standardization is better," the illusions of full transparency, global interconnectedness, and so forth, these arguments are still vitally important. It is still too often suggested that the next technological fix is the only step lying between the messy present and achieving perfection at all the dimensions of the quality concept. Criticizing such rhetorics is crucial, if only because of the disillusion that will surely come when the fix is embraced—when it is discovered that technologies do not solve problems, but merely displace them. Yet something deeply important is missing when the analysis stops here. The fact that the goals of the current reformers show much continuity with those of their predecessors does not mean that there is no simultaneous *transformation* occurring in their aims. The fact that we are still talking about standardization does not mean that we are now not speaking about some very different issues and tensions as we were, say, twenty years ago.

In addition, this criticism ultimately avoids dealing with the very issues that motivate the quality protagonists. By showing that many uses of terms such as *effectiveness* and *efficiency* can be easily deconstructed, the urgency to improve the effectiveness and efficiency of medical care is ironicized. The politics of this critique lie in the debunking of the rationalist drive and in the demonstration of the hidden work required to perform evidence-based medicine. Conveniently, however, the question whether there is not indeed something deeply suboptimal or wrong in the current health care system is sidestepped. Yet when it is important to give voice to the doctors, nurses, and patients who have to do all this hidden work, why is it not equally or more crucial to consider how more effectiveness or efficiency—however performed— can be beneficial to patients, nurses, and/or doctors? Put more dramatically, we may criticize the committee's analysis of Western health care as overly ambitious, reductive, and so forth, but can we fail to deal with these problems completely? We can debunk the committee's analysis of the death toll of medical errors—pointing at the unclear definitions, the questionable comparison between safety-critical industries such as air travel and medicine—but can we avoid addressing the problems of unnecessary deaths and organizational failure at all?[10]

All the stories in this book are about rendering practices more scientific, objective, transparent, and so forth. We could have told all these stories as attempts to replace disorder by (an ultimately elusive) order, to create a new network, to discipline medical work in and through introducing standards. This book could have been yet another story about standardization in medicine as a unilinear process with a singular outcome—standardized medicine. Yet standardized medicine, evidence-based medicine, and objectivity are not so much qualifiers that we can have more or less of. If we look closer, if we take the time to let ourselves be surprised about the varieties inside and between these developments, we constantly encounter *different universalities*. Whether we study novel record-keeping standards, the emergence of evidence-based medicine, or measures of risk control, we are struck by the fact that the differences we encounter—that are rarely discussed—are as relevant as the continuities that we always hear about. Our study of standardizing medicine, then, is a study of how different definitions of risk and of objectivity struggle to become prominent; how evidence-based medicine becomes appropriated and reappropriated by medical students, by health care professionals, and by professions as a whole; and how what "patient-centered" means is decided.

Consequently, the politics of standards does not lie in the debate whether standards bring quality of care *or* dehumanization, professional autonomy *or* deprofessionalization. Rather, the politics of standards lies in elucidating the specificities of the socio-material networks that emerge. We want to decipher, then, what patient, what notion of medical work, what objectivity, what configuration of professionals, third parties, regulators, and so forth is constituted by a specific standard—in a specific practice. How a safe medical practice is established—and at what costs. At a basic level, it is obvious that the many goals to be enhanced through standardization often clash. Although it argues that "for the most part, the six [dimensions of quality listed above] are complementary and synergistic," the *Quality Chasm* report recognizes that "at times however, there will be tensions among them."[11] Patient-centeredness and effectiveness, for example, might be in tension when patients are refused straws of hope because they are "not proven." Likewise, efficiency might be at odds with both patient-centeredness and effectiveness. Some of the more rigorous utilization review practices are a case in point. Being fully oriented toward patients, informing them, supporting them, guiding them through the individual steps and organizing the care system around their needs will generally be more costly than simply demanding from them that they follow the logic most efficient for the specific health care function you operate. Similarly, putting the medical state of the art into practice often implies treating many patients who were not treated before, more comprehensively, and starting earlier in their illness trajectories. This may be more effective, but it will definitely not reduce the overall costs of the health care system—at least not in the short run.

More important, we focused on how what *counts* as effectiveness or patient-centeredness can differ. The insurance physicians' standards were about the struggle to define the very meaning of objectivity and the validity of different types of evidence. We emphasised how different standards produce different worlds: changing intra- and interprofessional relations, changing the very meaning of professional autonomy, and distributing risk in different ways over different actors. A "safe" thalidomide was created at a highly specific cost, we showed in Chapter 5. Safety is not one simple thing; its achievement can take many different forms. The quest for accountability, likewise, is not simply driven by or facilitated through more standards. Just what accountability should look like, whose burden it is to carry it and whose to demand it, what information should satisfy this request, and so forth are the very conflicts that are *settled* in and through the creation of standards. It is such differences that we have to focus on. It is in this way that we can start to tackle the issues about errors in medicine, unnecessary deaths, and organizational dysfunctioning without having to take over the illusion of unequivocal evidence, a single effectiveness, or a contradiction-free efficiency.[12]

We argue, then, that the committee's aims—a health care service that is more effective, efficient, patient-centered, safe, timely, and equitable—are too important to merely ironicize. We argue, likewise, that standardization is not only a phenomenon we want to study and hopefully influence. We feel that procedural standards can play a core role in addressing these issues. In Chapter 2 we argued that procedural standards are coordinating tools which, when properly articulated with the local expertise of health care workers, can enhance competencies of workers, articulate care processes more smoothly, facilitate the execution of highly complex diagnostic and treatment schemes, and so forth. Western health care practices are currently far from effective, efficient, patient-centered, safe, timely, and equitable—however exactly defined—not so much because of the failings of *individual* health care workers, but because of a lack of coordination of their individual activities. Work around individual patient trajectories is fragmented because of intra- and interorganizational borders that have much relation with the organizations' and professions' histories, but little with the needs of individual patients. Tasks are not aligned; organizational routines do not articulate with each other; information is not shared. The social organization of medical work still emphasizes the importance of mastery through individual experience; there is still little stimulus toward incorporating new insights in one's practice routines.[13]

All this implies, then, that the issue is not *whether* procedural standardization is good or possible, but *how* it should be done. The issue is not for or against evidence-based medicine, guidelines, or electronic patient records, but *what* shape they should take and *how* they should be put to work. A focus on the multiple goals and interests at stake and on the way standards have to be made to work is of vital importance here. A deep knowledge of the characteristics of health care work is crucial to be able to find the synergy between the standard's coordinating activity and the staff members' embodied expertise. Similarly, a thorough understanding of the different worlds aligned and transformed in any standardization process is a sine qua non for any such process to be successful. Successful, here, means to contribute to the needs of both individual professionals and patients and organizations; to align these wherever possible rather than offset them against each other. This definition is neither complete nor fully realizable—it will have to be amended for any specific problem to be addressed. But this definition does put our commitment to be *part of* rather than above the networks we study at center stage.

A DIFFERENT STANDARDIZATION:
AWAY FROM SIMPLE SOLUTIONS

What, then, if anything, *is* different about the current calls for quality improvement as exemplified in the committee's report? Of all the potential benefits that coordinating tools could bring, the current focus on evidence-based guidelines has resulted in preciously little. Evidence-based guidelines are mainly designed to inform individual physicians about the state-of-the-art knowledge—a rather minimal form of coordination to begin with. Confronted with the overload of guidelines all competing for attention—Wiener refers to 24,000 guidelines in operation in 1995 in the United States alone[14]—physicians more often than not see guidelines as just another piece of information. Generally speaking, compliance with guidelines is minimal, we observed in Chapter 3. The coordinating potential of such tools is thereby reduced to linking all professionals receiving these mailings together in a collective vaguely oriented to enhancing evidence-based modes of working. This serves some goals at the level of the professions—but it hardly makes a difference at the level of the work these professionals do.

In the chapter on applying evidence to health care practice, the committee's report underwrites the conclusion now also broadly accepted within the guidelines community that "the dissemination of guidelines alone has not been a very effective method of improving clinical practice."[15] Interestingly, the report here not merely points to the many supplementary implementation measures as a solution. A plethora of behavioral, social-psychological, and marketing techniques are currently drawn upon and tested to see how physicians can be motivated to change their practice routines. Yet it is not the *mind* of the physician that should be the ultimate focus of attention. The massive enterprise of guideline implementation activities is all too singularly focused on overcoming this one, resistant barrier to the diffusion of optimal knowledge. After all, as the social studies of science and technology tell us, knowledge is not merely in the head. Transforming medical decision criteria or ways to handle a diagnosis or therapy implies transforming the whole practice in which these criteria are materially and organizationally embedded. Quoting Weed, the committee argues:

> Until now, we have believed that the best way to transmit knowledge from its source to its use in patient care is to first load the knowledge

into human minds . . . and then expect those minds, at great expense, to apply the knowledge to those who need it. However, there are enormous "voltage drops" along this transmission line for medical knowledge.[16]

With physicians being only one part of the network of health care delivery, and their heads already being rather overloaded, we couldn't agree more. Since knowledge is embedded in a practice's organizational routines, forms, protocols, and even working hierarchies,[17] embedding a guideline in the social and material context in which health care professionals function might be a much more fruitful way of getting guidelines to work.

More generally, the committee's reports have a refreshing focus on the health care *system* as the unit of analysis rather than the health care *professional*. For at least two decades, guidelines and other decision support techniques primarily focused on correcting what was seen as a core weakness of the health care delivery system: the individual professional's limited cognitive abilities.[18] For quite some time, the dominant discourse on the professional quality of medical work turned around judgmental errors, the individual's capacity to keep up with the literature, the doctor's failure to estimate probabilities, and so forth. These reports, however, state adamantly that it is utterly wrong to focus on the individual health care professional: the quality of the overall patient care trajectory is predominantly due to the way the overall *system* of actions and events hangs together. Strongly drawing on system theory, the reports state that it is through transforming the health care system, through altering the conditions in which health care professionals do their work, that the quality of their individual work will also increase. Rather than stressing the cognitive limitations or the economic drives of individual health care professionals, then, the *Quality Chasm* report includes a chapter on aligning payment policies with quality improvement, outlining just how several current payment methods have "perverse" effects. Fee-for-service schemes subsidize overuse, and can actually hamper incentives to improve care delivery when the improvement yields less patient contacts, for example. Budget-based approaches, on the other hand, can stimulate underuse, and similarly work against care innovation when potential savings, for example, threaten to be seen as a reason to lower the budget. In many ways, payment schemes actually stimulate individuals and organizations to deliver poor-quality health care.[19] Rather than focusing on the limitations of individual actors, the report focuses on the limitations in the way their actions interrelate and are coordinated and the ways current competencies are suboptimally drawn upon.

Similar to the aims of this book, then, the committee is concerned about the conditions in which health care professionals do their work. In significant parts, its view on professionals aligns with the depiction of knowledge workers in science and technology studies. The latter stress the importance of tacit knowledge and learning-in-practice, and, consequently, see the professional as the core potential innovative force in medicine. Professionals, after all, are most intimately involved in the complex core business of health care organizations. Health care innovation needs to take seriously the peculiarities of medical work and to build upon the professionals' drives in order for it to be successful.[20]

In addition, the report does state that the different dimensions of quality may clash. Although it remains a rather underdeveloped theme, the very notion that one's quality is not the same as another's is crucial. In any quality project the questions who gains what, who loses what, and which side effects are accepted or taken for granted are highly relevant. This becomes especially poignant, of course, where the future position of the medical profession and the individual professional is at stake. One core author of the report, Donald Berwick, has repeatedly argued for the importance of separating measurement for judgment from measurement for improvement.[21] The former is about measuring the quality of a medical practice (its clinical effectiveness, the satisfaction of patients, its efficiency, and so forth) with the aim of helping patients, payers, and others compare the performance of medical practices, or to assure to them that a minimal level of quality is guaranteed. This supposes that health care professionals' work should and can be fully transparent, and that customers and other stakeholders can freely pick the best care available. As these conditions are never achieved (and the analyses in this book would lead us to say that they can never be achieved), any attempt to create transparency in this way is suspiciously monitored by the profession, and leads to many defensive reactions (including the most creative ways of number-jostling imaginable).[22]

Alternatively, measurement for improvement presupposes that it is the involved health care professionals themselves who do the measuring in their own health care processes, reflect upon the outcomes, and

then attempt to improve the processes so as to improve the overall outcomes achieved. In this version of quality improvement, the professionals take the lead. They prove to the outside world that high-quality care
is their core concern and part and parcel of their work—rather than the
outside world trying to judge quality as if it is a feature that can be simply caught in a report figure or a list of mortality numbers.

The latter approach is centrally focused on care innovation, the core
role of the professional in this, and the contextual nature of information
about a practice's performance. It is this approach that lies most near
the insights gained in this book—and again, it is this approach that the
report emphasizes.[23] Yet this cannot be an exclusive choice. By embracing this approach, and by criticizing the illusionary idea that full transparency would be possible, one overlooks the fact that from the perspective of patients, even a rather blunt insight into the health care industry's
performance is better than nothing. Here different realizations of quality clash again. Patients might not know how exactly to judge detailed,
risk-adjusted mortality figures of coronary bypass surgery, for example.
Yet they might not care about the potential injustice done to individual
surgeons, nor might they care about the damage that these publications
might do to the willingness of health care professionals to reassess their
own work critically. They are now able to avoid the bottom half of the
list—that part where the mortality rates are several times higher than
those at the top of the list. Likewise, they may just be happy to learn
that these mortality figures decreased some 40 percent in the few years
after their first publication.[24]

As a final point, the report takes a refreshingly pragmatist approach
in laying out how better health care should be realized. Just as we emphasized the unpredictability of technological development, and the
mutual transformations of procedural standards and health care practices, the committee does not lay out a blueprint of some ideal health
care system or a step-by-step roadmap for getting from here to there.
Emphasizing the unpredictability of behavior in complex adaptive systems, the report argues for an approach that sets modest goals in an
iterative, incremental fashion, and that maximally draws upon the resources that happen to be available. Likewise, the measurements required to inform practical action are low key and as minimal and simple
as possible, rather than precise, detailed, and heavily standardized as in
any formal clinical trial.[25]

A DIFFERENT STANDARDIZATION:
MAKING PROCEDURAL STANDARDS WORK

How could procedural standards play a more significant role in Western health care? How can we draw more fruitfully upon procedural standards as coordinating tools? Just what could make the difference between yet another failed standardization project and a care innovation that makes a difference? How can we differentiate between standardization for standardization's sake and "smart" standardization? To conclude this book, we discuss several lessons learned that are a first step to answering these questions.

1. The potential synergy between procedural standards and professional work can only be found in a careful unraveling of care processes, a redistribution of work activities over the different professionals and the patient, and the use of the coordinating tool to (help) make this redistribution and subsequent interrelation of tasks possible.

In Chapter 1 we saw how even the introduction of a simple technology such as the patient-centered record transformed not only the individual professional's working practices, but ultimately affected the overall system, including the system of professions[26] and the architecture of hospital buildings. Rather than attempting to diffuse a technology, and then being confronted with the organizational transformations that will necessarily follow, it is much more fruitful to draw upon a procedural standard as *one aspect* of a socio-technical change process, in which the whole practice is redesigned.[27] We can only take advantage of the potential benefits of coordinating technologies when we thoroughly reconsider how current work practices could be reorganized. Similarly, it is meaningless to try to enhance cooperation between individual's work activities without pondering about the way these work activities may be transformed in their interrelation. Their embedded logics might be more tied to individual preferences or organizational histories than to an aim to produce quality (however it is defined). Moreover, when taken together, their individual logics might interact in ways that are suboptimal at the system level.

Let us discuss a real example, taken from the American context, but sadly universal in its implications. When Ruth found out she was pregnant, she went to her primary care physician for a referral to a neighborhood birth center. She had to schedule the appointment with her physician during work hours, quite inconveniently because she did not want to let her boss know she was pregnant. On the day of the appointment, she first registered with the receptionist and then saw her physician. The primary care physician confirmed the pregnancy with a urine test, similar to the one Ruth used to find out she was pregnant, and then wrote the referral letter. Ruth called for an appointment with the birth center and was able to secure a spot on a Saturday morning. She presented herself with the referral letter to the birth center's receptionist, who placed the letter in a file folder she retrieved from the archive behind her. Ruth met with the midwife, answered a ten-page list of questions to assess any risk factors during pregnancy, and underwent a physical exam. Ruth would have preferred to answer the survey at home because she would have been able to consult with her own mother about her family's reproductive history.

The midwife ordered that a blood sample be drawn and, according to the new hospital policy, suggested that Ruth undergo a genetic test for cystic fibrosis. The receptionist prepared the referral forms and sent Ruth to the blood laboratory in the nearby hospital. Ruth again registered in the main hospital and then waited for a phlebotomist to draw the blood. Because it was a Saturday, the phlebotomist was unable to draw the blood for the cystic fibrosis genetic test. Ruth would have to come back during the week.

In this example, even though pregnancy checkups are routine events, all steps need to be planned and executed one at a time, resulting in an inefficient use of patients' and health care providers' time and a chance for misunderstandings and suboptimal care. Because it was too difficult to take time off work and after weighing the risks, for example, Ruth decided to forego the cystic fibrosis genetic test.

Now, imagine an outpatient clinic where the receptionist contacts a patient at home to figure out the reason for the visit. Relying on a simple decision support system, the receptionist determines whether the patient qualifies for a predefined standard patient trajectory. If the patient qualifies, the receptionist can already plan a number of blood laboratory tests and ask additional questions. She could forward the questionnaire used to assess the pregnancy risks. The receptionist can then enter the answers to those questions and the tests in the patient information system and make them available to the subsequent health care providers.

The information system could also contain standardized care plans for more highly trained health care providers, for example, in the form of predefined therapeutic interventions that can be activated with a click of a mouse. When presented as templates that can be easily modified, they structure the professional's work in a helpful way, allowing fast access to routine action-paths, while fully retaining the flexibility to adjust these plans to individual trajectories when necessary. In Ruth's case, one adaptation would be that she intended to give birth in a birth center and work with midwifes instead of in a hospital with an OB/GYN as is typical in the United States.

The planning of all the links in the chain can be further supported via collaborative agenda systems, to plan as many activities as possible in a convenient time frame. Instead of spreading four different visits over several weeks, a pregnant patient could visit a primary care physician, a nurse-midwife, a phlebotomist, and a genetic counselor in one morning and end up with a care plan at the end.

There are many variations possible to this simple example, within or between health care organizations, more or less integrating care and cure, and more or less organized around specific patient categories or groups. In some instances, it may be possible to have the patient play a central, active role in the care process. Diabetes patients, for example, would be able to monitor and adjust their own therapeutic regimes to a far greater extent than currently. The common denominator is the integration of a professionally optimal mode of handling patients (a guideline) into a work practice redesigned so as to optimally perform this guideline. In this way, the guideline becomes truly and flexibly embedded in the organizational and informational structure of the work itself.

   2. Use standardization where it enhances competencies and qualities rather than reduces them.

In the alternative scenario, receptionists and nurses receive new tasks and responsibilities in the care process: backed up by decision support techniques (including detailed guidelines) they are allowed to take up a central role and take over some of the specialists' tasks. The overall quality of the care delivery is guaranteed by those professionals who helped design the decision support techniques and take care of patients who fall outside the standard modules. Whenever uncertainty remains (whether patients qualify for the protocols and support techniques, for example), patients are directly referred to that specialist.

The specialists' work is standardized only when they enter the patient in a standardized care program—and these programs can still be adapted at any point. The simple decision support programs and practice guidelines that afford a new role for the receptionist and streamline the care process would generate an unworkable level of standardization for more highly trained health care providers. Specialists would continuously need to over-rule the system's advice, spend too much time on trying to work with (and around) the system, and might eventually lose their motivation. The history of medical information systems has shown that the road toward autonomous or intelligent decision-making systems has been a dead-end street.[28] It makes more sense to search for the optimal synergy between professionals' knowledge and the system's capacities rather than have them compete. It makes more sense, in other words, to build "intelligence" into the care process than into the standardized information technology.[29]

In redesigning care processes, standardization should thus be localized in only some specific parts of the health care process (e.g., routine diagnostic tests, repeated aspects of therapeutic trajectories, recurring triage moments, etc.). In other aspects of the health care process, possible variation should be embraced. This ensures that competency and quality are maximally optimized throughout the entire health care process. Highly trained specialists would focus primarily on the patients who fall outside the standard trajectories, on the linkages between the standardized elements of the care process, and on fine tuning the individual diagnostic and therapeutic tasks.

In this way, it would also no longer mainly be the "most highly trained professional . . . with the greatest opportunity cost [who ends up] in the data-entry role."[30] When the health care process is restructured so that the secretary, nurse practitioners, and the patients themselves enter data in a standardized way, a much more complete file becomes feasible without any individual care professional carrying too large a burden. When the follow-up is subsequently appropriately reorganized as well, clinical outcomes may be registered, and aggregated data may be used for feedback to the overall group of professionals involved in the health care process. Through such standardization, moreover, subsequent information handling or coordination tasks by the patient care information system are made possible—such as alerts or reminders,[31] semi-automatic letters, and so forth.

3. "Flexible standards" is not a contradiction in terms.

An important characteristic of standards is their flexibility. In the alternative scenario the specialist could easily deviate from the standardized care plan and quickly make adaptations. A standardized protocol's strength depends on the extent that the tool allows for deviation and improvisation. Flexibility implies that the system is not more detailed than required, not more stringent than necessary, not more imperative than usable. A flexible procedural standard can be smoothly integrated in daily health care work. It implies not detailing thirty steps when three suffice, no choice of 5,000 diagnostic categories when 400 are sufficient.

Flexibility also implies that the standard can be easily revised and adapted to local demands or to new scientific insights.[32] Compared to Danish GP systems, for example, the coding schemes used in British primary care systems are easily adaptable, rendering the entire system more meaningful and acceptable to GPs.[33] In addition, it should be possible to adapt standard care paths to newly emerging insights and knowledge, for example, based on feedback from aggregated health data tabulated from the support systems themselves.

This might sound obvious and simple but it is not. The importance of local adaptability, for example, clashes with the demand that a standard is just that: *standard*. Everywhere applicable, everywhere similar. And simple, pragmatic standards that do not standardize more than necessary might lead to an unwieldy patchwork of overlapping and contradictory standards. Many standard developers abhor such disorder, and much effort is spent on attempts to develop (inter)national, all-encompassing models in which data, decision criteria, and work processes are ordered in formal, unequivocal, and universal ways. Both within several European countries and at the European level, many resources have been wasted on attempts to create the ultimate model of the health care process.[34] Likewise, much work has been fruitlessly invested in the quest for a modern Tower of Babel to resolve the vagueness and multiplicity of medical language.[35] Such standards are inevitably very elaborate and complex, and contain a logic opaque to everyone except the designers themselves. Because these standards are so far removed from daily practice, they become difficult to implement and lead to manifold frictions in the care work. And once those standards are implemented, finally, they are very rigid and hard to change. Any proposed alteration of the complex whole has to be carefully investigated for its consistency and logic; any such proposition has to follow a long trajectory of (inter)national consultation rounds and committee meetings.[36]

4. Search for the exception to the rule: reduce standardization in the health care process by optimally drawing upon procedural standards.

Drawing upon the functionality of procedural standards without obstructing actual work processes is thus possible by (1) searching for the right parts of the work to standardize and (2) opting for flexible standards. In addition, procedural standards may sometimes allow for an actual *reduction* of standardization. First of all, in many of the examples given above, tasks were redelegated among the different team members so that more highly trained professionals in fact ended up doing *less* standard tasks. Clerical personnel could take over more administrative tasks, or fill in patient questionnaires and patients themselves could enter monitoring data. Similarly, properly supported nurse practitioners could easily handle many of the more routine patient visits, so that specialist physicians could concentrate on those cases that truly require their expertise.

In these instances, the overall level of standardization may still increase, while it is more appropriately distributed over the team members involved. (Lest we are misunderstood: not leading to *more* standardization for lesser trained professionals and clerks, but to new competencies and changed job descriptions.) These are examples in which the well-known thesis that standardization (the coming of guidelines, protocols, external accountability) necessarily leads to a mechanization of work (and thus a concurrent loss of clinical autonomy) is clearly refuted (see also Chapter 4).

In addition, procedural standards may make a redesign of work practices realizable so that an actual *overall* reduction of standardization becomes possible. An interdisciplinary team working at different times of the day in different locales requires an intense tuning of schedules and work practices to diagnose and treat a patient as a team. How are tasks split up? Who does what? How does person A inform person B? In such a situation, the coordination of work depends crucially on joint procedural standards and interdisciplinary patient records. Drawing upon information technology, such a work practice might be reorganized so that professionals coordinate their actions no longer *asynchronously* but *synchronously*, through the data immediately accessible in a joint data set.[37] In this way, this interdisciplinary team could do without much of the standardization required for the intricate coordination between their separate activities. Rather, they could draw upon roughly sketched care plans that are filled in on the spot in the direct interaction between the professionals. The coordination tasks, in this example, are handed back to professionals, which has become feasible (and efficient) because the overall complexity of the coordination job (linking the separated actions) has been minimized. These care professionals could also have free access to each other's agenda, so that they could easily adjust the care paths to the particular demands of individual patient trajectories.

These latter examples are hard to find in current health care practice. This is not unexpected: standardization, we said earlier, is still too often perceived as a good in and of itself. To employ procedural standards to actually *increase* the decision space of care providers or to *reduce* overall standardization remains counterintuitive. In the light of the specific nature of medical work, however, this may be an overlooked strategy.

5. The success of such a redesign of the care process is crucially dependent on the opportunities given to the professionals (and other users) to skillfully integrate the tool's demands in their work practices.

Even for simple triage situations as described above (the outpatient clinic secretary categorizing a pregnant patient), decision support systems, when left to their own devices, are remarkably ineffective. Worried patients end up worrying more, and the tool's answers more often than not fail to answer the question as the patient phrased it.[38] To translate between patient and tool requires interpretation by the secretary—and knowledge about what the tool's purpose is, and what the meaning of the preset categories is. Similarly, paramedics responsible for a diagnostic pretrajectory should be able to react properly to a patient whose situation is such that a test is unlikely to provide clinically relevant information. It requires much skill to act appropriately in such situations: knowledge about the test's purposes and clinical skills to realize its inappropriateness.

For the potential synergy between procedural standards and professional work to emerge, then, the tool's coordination tasks should not be seen as self-sufficient. In the common parlance of "intelligent agents" and "computerized carepaths," this imperative is easily forgotten. Yet we already concluded that constantly bridging the needs of the patient or the work situation and the tool's functionality is a highly skilled activity. It is crucial that the secretary, the paramedics, and other users are supported in this task: through formal training, but also through the constant opportunity to learn from and interact with the other actors in the care chain. Such lateral connections between individuals that hold seemingly independent positions in the formal workflow are essential to facilitate this articulation work.[39] This comes down to facilitating physical access to each other, and enhancing unstructured modes of communication, such as e-mail or telephone.[40] When the procedural standard controls the work process so rigidly that the receptionist is no longer in touch with the specialist, then the former will fail to grasp just what the triage aims to do. Their tasks are formally separated: according to a workflow diagram, these two individuals need not be in direct personal contact with one another. But without adequate and not overly structured contacts between the two, they lose an opportunity to inform and learn from each other. These are simple things that may seem insignificant in the light of the larger organizational changes that the procedural standard brings. Yet they make the difference between being able or not being able to integrate the standard's functionality in the ongoing flow of work. Thereby, they make the difference between a tool that clashes with that flow of work, or a tool that lifts professionals' work to a higher level.

RETURN TO UTSTEIN

A dozen years after the leading international emergency researchers gathered in Utstein to standardize what counted as properly recorded first aid life-saving behavior, the quest for more and better standards in medicine is only becoming stronger. Our book has shown what these standardization attempts amount to: how they are not primarily about flushing the breath of life out of medicine but about creating new worlds, potentially richer and more multidimensional as any less standardized world can ever be. As coordinating devices in an ever more complex health care system, procedural standards are becoming ever more important. Concurrently, it becomes ever more important to see them as the world making entities that they are, and to scrutinize just how they redefine patient-hood, working relationships, clinical autonomy, risk distributions, and so forth.

At the same time, the topic we focused on is transforming itself while we speak. From a search for practice guidelines that transfer scientific knowledge to individual physicians who do not adequately keep up with the literature, evidence-based medicine has developed itself as an overall *attitude*, scorning experience-based knowledge and demanding hard (meaning: randomized clinical trial-based) evidence. As a concurrent movement, quality improvement[41] now seems to be taking over the momentum that is currently seeping out of the singular emphasis on guideline development and its implementation efforts. In doing so, it is reviving many of the tropes behind most previous standardization movements: an emphasis on efficiency, effectiveness, safety, and central attention to the patient. Yet in interesting ways, this recent development seems to have learned from some of the limitations of earlier efforts. It is more oriented toward the way health care practices as *collectives* produce certain health outcomes, rather than focusing (and implicitly blaming) individual practitioners. It stresses the fact that quality is a multidimensional concept—and that these dimensions may not harmoniously interact. It emphasizes the active role of rank-and-file professionals in quality improvement projects—explicitly preferring local initiatives and commitment, with its concurrent patchy and incremental change patterns, to global change programs that promise sweeping, "big bang" revolutions. Finally, it warns against overly technocratic attempts to steer and compare health care practices through an overly simplistic trust in aggregate numbers.

We are not uncritically embracing this movement. We readily confess that this is a rather optimistic and selective reading of the quality improvement literature. Yet our point is that a productive dialogue *with* these heirs of the standardization movements is called for, and possible. Entering into debate with the subjects of this study, so to speak, is what is now most relevant, much more so than reiterating the persisting dominance of elusive rationalization rhetoric to our own home audience—critical social scientists, science and technology scholars, and so forth. In this development, which constantly reinvents itself, and which never speaks with one, simple voice, differences *can* be made through a feed-back of some of our home audience's insights into this playing field. This is how the previous section's five points should be read: as our attempt to do politics through standardization. To explicate the ways in which procedural standards can bring forward livable worlds. This, in our view, is an important way in which we can breathe life back into sociology's dealing with standardization. It is not medicine whose life needs to be saved from the onslaught of standardization: it is the so-cial sciences whose standardization critiques are becoming deadly stale. Failing to redraw our own politics of standardization would not only render us blind to all the transformations that are occurring in front of us. It would also render us powerless in its further development: doomed to just bemoan the further "McDonaldization" of medicine, and the dehumanization of patient care.

Notes

INTRODUCTION

1. Cummins et al. 1991.
2. Eisenberg et al. 1990b.
3. Eisenberg et al. 1990a, 1249.
4. Cummins et al. 1991.
5. Becker 1993, 2.
6. Shear and Maser 1994.
7. Miller et al. 1995.
8. Kossoff and Nyborg 1989.
9. Turnberg 1997.
10. Sackett and Rosenberg 1995.
11. Field and Lohr 1990.
12. Woolf et al. 1996, 947.
13. The blood test actually checks for the antibodies to the virus; see the fact-sheet of the NIH at www. niaid.nih.gov/factsheets/stdherp.htm.
14. See http://www.infopoems.com for more information.
15. See the vitriolic tone of the "focused issue" of the journal, volume 3 (2), April 1997. Incidentally, the critics are also critical of medical sociology. One of them states that "doctor's envy" and "anti-medical prejudice" is the foundational principle of sociology of health and illness (Charlton 1997b, 95).
16. Jackson and Feder 1998.
17. Korcok 1994; Liang 1992; Rosser et al. 2001.
18. This clearinghouse will include any guideline that is systematically developed, evidence-based, and created or updated within the past five years. The guidelines have to be "produced under the auspices of medical specialty associations; relevant professional societies, public or private organizations, government agencies at the Federal, State, or local level; or health care organizations or plans." Given these relatively wide inclusion criteria, the actual number of guidelines included (921) is low; this might be due to the fact that the guidelines have to be submitted by the original guideline developers.
19. Woolf et al. 1999.
20. Pearson 1992.
21. Krislov 1997, 12–16.
22. O'Connell 1993.

23. Morgan 1989; Shenhav 1999; Chandler 1977.

24. Beniger 1986.

25. Shenhav 1999.

26. Ibid., 63.

27. Morgan 1989.

28. Ibid.

29. Ibid., 14.

30. Miles et al. 1997, 83.

31. Drury 1922, 77.

32. While Taylor aimed to triple and quadruple production rates, he cautioned against too big salary increases. The salary increases needed to be "substantial," but getting rich too quickly decreased productivity. He aimed for salary increases of 60 percent (Taylor 1914, 74).

33. Ibid., 130.

34. Noble 1984, 33.

35. Ibid., 34.

36. Drury 1922, 35–39.

37. Gilbreth quoted in Graham 1998, 74.

38. Krislov 1997, 48.

39. Ibid., 52.

40. Grindley 1995.

41. Coles 1949; Williamson 1992.

42. Dickersin and Manheimer 1998. Whether Cochrane is a true predecessor of evidence-based medicine is up for debate. Both the EBM camp and their critics claim Cochrane as an inspiration for their cause. See Marshall 1997.

43. Wennberg 1999.

44. Wennberg 1984. See also Belkin 1997 for a more conspirational history.

45. Field and Lohr 1990, 21.

46. Brook 1989, 80.

47. Manning 2002.

48. Dickersin and Manheimer 1998, 327.

49. Ornstein et al. 1992.

50. Santucci et al. 1990; Laires et al. 1995; Dick et al. 1997.

51. Rodwin 2001, 439.

52. Geyman 1999.

53. Berkwitz 1998.

54. Charlton 1997a, 169.

55. Miles et al. 1997, 84.

56. Charlton 1997a, 169.

57. Rosoff 2001, 327.

58. Ritzer 1992.

59. Strading and Davies 1997.

60. Charlton 1997b, 87.

61. Brunsson and Jacobsson 2000, 172.

62. Bowker and Star 1999; Krislov 1997; Grindley 1995; Brunsson and Jacobsson 2000.

63. The latest edition of the *Handbook of Medical Sociology* (Bird et al. 2000) contains several calls to study guidelines and evidence-based medicine but no empirical studies (but cf. Green and Britten 1998).

64. Haraway 1991.

65. Timmermans 1999a.

66. Latour 1999.

67. Berg 1997b.

68. Berg and Mol 1998.

69. Foucault 1973.

70. Hacking 1999, 125.

71. Hacking 1998.

72. Epstein 1996; Epstein in press.

73. Cummins et al. 1991, 963.

74. Becker 1993.

75. Ritzer and Walczak 1988.

76. WWWebster Dictionary.

77. Williamson 1992.

78. For a discussion of such standards, see Schmidt and Werle 1998.

79. For a discussion of terminological standardization, see Bowker and Star 1999.

80. Schmidt and Werle 1998.

81. Shapiro 1997.

82. Ginsburg 1998.

83. Influenced by Keynesian economics and the Depression, the gold standard was abandoned in the 1930s in favor of monetary standards. The economic gold standard thus evolved. Similarly, we show, do medical "gold" standards.

84. Pellegrino 1996.

85. Aronowitz 1998, 26.

86. Yet see Pasveer 1992; Latour 1987a.

87. Glaser and Strauss 1967.

Chapter 1. Standardization in Medicine in the Twentieth Century

1. Bottomley 1918, 220.

2. Howell 1989, 1.

3. Rosenberg 1987; Stevens 1989.

4. Rosenberg 1987.

5. The Mayo Clinic was unique in that it was a group practice—yet even here all records were kept individually.

6. Quoted in Kurland and Molgaard 1981, 58.

7. Kurland and Molgaard 1981; Reiser 1978.

8. Craig 1990.

9. What exactly this science would be, however, was far from clear. See, for example, Rosenberg 1987; Vogel and Rosenberg 1979; Warner 1985.

10. Rosenberg 1987.

11. See, for example, Pasveer (1989) and Cartwright (1995) for histories of visualization technologies in medicine

12. Craig 1989–90; Howell 1995.

13. Bottomley 1918, 220.

14. Foucault 1973; Porter 1997.

15. Klazinga 1997; Mol and van Lieshout 1989.

16. Bottomley 1918, 219.

17. Rosenberg 1987; Stevens 1989.

18. Mansholt 1931.

19. Starr 1982.

20. Codman et al. 1914, 73. In these days, surgery was a blossoming enterprise: with the emergence of antisepsis and analgesics, the number (and kinds) of operations performed within hospitals exploded (and with that the profile of the surgeon) (Porter 1997; Lawrence 1992).

21. Codman et al. 1914, 71.

22. Kurland and Molgaard 1981; Reiser 1978.

23. Kilgore 1915, 767.

24. Hughes 1932.

25. Fee splitting occurred when a physician referred a patient to the specialist. The specialist would split the fee with the referring physician, generating a potential conflict of interest.

26. Hughes 1932, 96.

27. *Yearbook of the American College of Surgeons 1919*, cited in Atwater 1989, 62.

28. Reiser 1984, 1991a, 1991b.

29. Anonymous 1914; cf. Slobe 1923, 63.

30. Reverby 1981; Reiser 1984.

31. Dr. Homer Gage, discussant in Bottomley 1918, 221

32. Atwater 1989; Stevens 1989; Long and Golden 1989; Lynaugh 1989.

33. Howell 1995.

34. In a 1921 American Hospital Association list of reasons for keeping clinical records, however, providing "the attending staff with a written record of the patient's progress" still ranks only fifth! (Bachmeyer 1922b).

35. Craig 1989–90, 1990.

36. Mannix 1935; Brotherhood 1913.

37. Stevens 1919, 324.

38. Huffman 1972, 6th edition, 21, quoting an editorial in the May 1919 issue of *Hospital Management*.

39. Craig 1989–90, 63.

40. Ibid.; Yates 1989; Clapesettle 1954.

41. Stevens 1989, 324.

42. Actor-network theory, one of the dominant theoretical sources in the sociology of science and technology, stresses how these networks are always heterogeneous, that is, made up of humans and things. Actor-network theory also stresses the importance and active role of objects in understanding the development of science, technology, and society. For introductory texts on actor-network theory, see Latour 1987a and Callon 1987. For a recent overview, see Law and Hassard 1999 and Latour 1999a.

43. See Warner 1986 on the still persistent importance of the principle of specificity in this period.

44. Rosenberg 1987, 309.

45. Davis 1920.

46. Lewinski-Corwin 1922, 604.

47. Brough 1935, 63.

48. Mayo 1919, cited in Reiser 1984, 311.

49. Lewinski-Corwin 1922, 604. In an investigation of sixty-six hospitals in 1935, 80 percent of the hospitals reported handling private and ward records in the same manner. Yet even at that time the resistances against this erasure of differences can be read from the statistics:

In 8 hospitals (15.6 percent) private patients' records are kept in the central record room and handled as ward records, with the following differences: . . . Private records are stamped "private" and are never used for study in 1 hospital. They are used only when permitted by the attending doctor in 3 hospitals. The blood Wassermann report is not placed on private records in 1 hospital. A few records of psychiatric cases are not placed in the central record file in 1 hospital. Records of "courtesy staff" patients are not included in the central record room in 1 hospital. A separate file is maintained for private patients' records in 2 hospitals (4 percent). (Stokes et al. 1933, 91)

50. Stevens 1919, 325.

51. Hughes 1932, 96.

52. Stevens 1919, 326.

53. Howell 1995.

54. Pearl 1921, 187.

55. Brough 1935, 63.

56. Auchincloss 1989 (1926), 307.

57. Stokes et al. 1933.

58. Bachmeyer 1922a; Smith 1913; Olsen 1920.

59. Kilgore 1915.

60. Anonymous 1912, 805.

61. Whiting Myers 1932, 64.

62. Anonymous 1904, 980.
63. Anonymous 1933, 82.
64. Smith 1990.
65. Munger 1928, 99–104.
66. Stevens 1919, 324.
67. Bugbee 1932, 1935.
68. Anonymous 1929c.
69. Genevieve Morse 1934, 99.
70. Mansholt 1931, 35. Author's translation from Dutch.
71. Bottomley 1918, 220.
72. Anonymous 1929b; Nortington Gamble 1989.
73. Schoute 1925, 112.
74. Mansholt 1931.
75. Ibid., 28–42.
76. Ibid.
77. Anonymous 1924; Anonymous 1929a.
78. Schoute 1925, 110. The extent of the Dutch physicians' opposition to schematism becomes even more evident when one realizes that even the most stark scientific management reformers stopped short of standardizing the content of medical work. Standardization may affect record-keeping procedures, nursing tasks, and the type of gloves and antiseptic to be used during surgery (cf. Doane 1931), and it may put in place minimal demands as to the education of doctors—but the making of the diagnosis or the performance of the surgical procedure itself remained untouched in the U.S. situation as well.
79. Anonymous 1916, 634; see Commissie in zake medische statistiek 1916.
80. Simon Schaffer quoting Maxwell in Wise 1995, 222.
81. Kilgore 1915.
82. Star and Ruhleder 1996; Hanseth et al. 1996.
83. Krislov 1997.
84. Anonymous 1929c, 68.
85. Mannix 1935, 71.
86. Howell 1989.
87. The reaction of the Dutch Medical Association is telling in this regard, as is the following remark, made in passing, by a hospital superintendent:

All institutions of any importance have striven to comply with the requirements of the American College of Surgeons, and in some hospitals the administration has, in doing so, kept records up to a higher standard than their medical staffs were prepared to appreciate or utilize. This is the only fault, in my opinion, in this tremendous helpful work. The fact is, that failure to gain approval by the college falls much more heavily upon the hospital than on the individual physician on its staff. (Munger 1928, 99).

88. Bottomley 1918, 220.
89. Schmidt and Werle 1998.

90. Bijker and Law 1992; Latour 1996.

91. This development is detailed in Berg and Harterink (2003). In the emergence of this modern patient, the introduction of the patient-centered record was of course only one important development among others. It was not the only institutional device endowing individual patients with a legally valid and retraceable personal history. The central record room, where the medical records were now to be stored, became a node in a much larger spanning web of "other hospitals, medical schools, pension bureaus, insurance companies, the industrial accident boards, workmen's compensation organizations and, by no means least, the department of public health" (Whiting Myers 1932, 66). All these institutions kept records, exchanged information, and produced persons as individuals with personal rights and personal histories of risks and disability, who were equal for the law and for the bureaucracies that counted, classified, and regulated them (Bowker and Star 1999).

CHAPTER 2. STANDARDS AT WORK

1. Reiser 1978, 140–41.

2. Field and Lohr 1990, 26.

3. The FRAM case was studied through document analysis, and through interviews and participatory observation on an oncological ward in a Dutch research hospital where this protocol was being used. The insurance physicians' case was studied through document analysis (of the reporting forms used in eight different regional offices in particular) and through interviews with insurance physicians, their physician supervisors ("coordinating physicians"), and their general managers (the directors of regional offices of the administrative bodies). The interview fragments are coded by two letters; the first referring to the regional office; the second indicating whether the person interviewed was a general *M*anager, a *C*oordinating physician, or an insurance physician involved in claim *E*valuation.

4. There are clear similarities between our analysis and the theoretical framework of Mintzberg (1979); for a powerful later adaptation, see Groth 1999. These analyses take place at the level of the organization as a whole, however; they speak of standardization of work activities as a way in which an organization achieves its need to coordinate the different work tasks that it encompasses. Moreover, in our analysis we focus more empirically on the coordinating power of the standards themselves, thereby undoing some of the static categorizations that inevitably characterize sweeping overviews such as Mintzberg's. For one, we are interested here in standardization of the work tasks *of professionals*, which falls outside of these authors' framework: for them, professional work is standardized only through a standardization of the *skills* learned in training. Finally, the question as to the normative relevance of empirical *differences* in procedural standards is not a question these authors pose themselves, yet it is a leading drive for us.

5. Solberg 2000; Freeman and Sweeney 2001.

6. We do not make a principled distinction between guidelines and proto-cols, although some authors would argue that the latter are stricter than the for-mer. This might sometimes be the case, but exceptions abound and preferences change per professional group and per time period. For instance, the insurance physicians used the terms *guideline* and *protocol* and *standard* completely inter-changeably. At any rate, the term *guideline* is obviously picked to make proce-dural standards more amenable to care professionals. A novel term is *carepath* or *clinical pathway*, which is often used for the interdisciplinary description of concrete steps. When detailed, they are rather similar to the protocols we've studied here.

7. MOPP stands for a combination of drugs.

8. BCNU stands for a combination of drugs.

9. We discuss the content of their work and their social position in more detail in Chapter 4.

10. Latour 1986, 1994.

11. Smith 1990.

12. Smith 1990; Barrett 1988.

13. Through a "precomputation of task interdependencies" the standard "reduces the space of possibilities" of the entities that interrelate with it (Schmidt and Simone 1996, 174).

14. Suchman 1993; Berg 1997b; Mintzberg 1979.

15. Shapiro 1997.

16. Epstein 1996; Löwy 1997.

17. Knorr-Cetina 1999; Keating and Cambrosio 2000.

18. Schmidt and Werle 1998, 4.

19. The so-called handshake protocol is the audible exchange of signals be-tween faxes at the beginning of a transmission, in which specific properties of the two involved machines are exchanged (such as the presence of error-correction, modem speed, etc.).

20. Schmidt and Werle 1998, 4–5.

21. Berg 1997b; Timmermans 1999b.

22. 1995, 154; cf. Rogers 1993.

23. Ingelfinger 1973; Christakis and Rivara 1998.

24. American Heart Association 1990, 238.

25. May 1985; Sanders 1999, 119.

26. On this issue of domination, actor-network theory and social construc-tivist analyses have often produced similar tales. In Latour's classic *Science in Action*, the overall trope is the work and translations involved in the alignment of heterogeneous allies in an expanding network; in the classic studies of Pinch and Bijker, closure is reached through aligning relevant social groups (Latour 1987a; Pinch and Bijker 1984). Although these studies stress that closure is al-ways temporary and that a network is never rendered fully docile, the emer-gence of a stabilized technology or procedure depends on consensus, or on ren-

dering equivalent and stabilizing that which was different and untamed. Creating a standard, in these studies, would imply extending the network by enrolling and tying together more and more allies. As the central network builder gains strength, as the network tightens, the individual elements in the network are made increasingly docile. For such explications of actor-network theory, see Latour 1987 and Michel Callon 1991. For core examples of such studies, see Law 1987; O'Connell 1993. Perceptive critiques on this tendency of actor-network theory are Haraway 1994; Lee and Brown 1994; Mol and Law 1994.

27. In Leigh Star's terms, guidelines are boundary objects (Star and Griesemer 1989).

28. But see the critical literature on the assumptions and realities of informed consent, beginning with, for example, Silverman 1987.

29. Every research protocol starts with summing up the inclusion and exclusion criteria for including patients.

30. Gomart and Hennion 1999; Latour 2003.

31. Attempting to control too tightly is unfeasible for many of the nonhuman elements as well: white-blood cells can behave erratically; X rays can show unexpected results; drugs can cause rare side effects; machines might break down. These are all matters which, when too tightly prescribed, would continually explode the meticulously prescribed path of the protocol. See also Hogle 1995; Singleton 1998.

32. Garfinkel 1967; Lynch 1993.

33. This example was given in the U.S. television program "60 Minutes" in a reportage of Leslie Stahl entitled: "How Many Does It Take to Change a Light Bulb in . . . ?" CBS television, 1994.

34. Knorr-Cetina 1999.

35. Benner 1984.

36. Smith 1978.

37. Wilkinson 1983; Zuboff 1988.

38. These are then not *quantitative* changes but *qualitative* ones: we are not talking about an increase or decrease in skills or control, but a *transformation* of the skills at stake.

39. Gasser 1986; Button and Harper 1993.

40. See Berg 1997a for a further critical discussion of the term *work arounds*. The work of Emilie Gomart (Gomart and Hennion 1999; Gomart 2003) has been very influential for the elaboration of this point.

41. Latour 1992; Knorr-Cetina 1999.

42. Berg 1997b.

43. Garfinkel 1967.

44. This chapter focused mainly on procedural standards. What about the other types of standards we discussed in the introduction? Do our notions of coordinating devices and active submission work for these standards as well? Without going into an elaborate discussion, it is clear that much of what has been said for procedural standards applies to terminological standards as well.

Working with preset categories or nomenclatures transforms the work of the individuals who draw upon them by outlining a set of concepts through which their activities are named, classified, and ordered.

Terminological standards differ from procedural standards in that they do not actively sequence tasks of individuals, or articulate tasks between individuals. Yet they form new communities of practitioners and align the activities of individuals by imposing common terminologies and categories. In this sense, terminological standards are coordinating devices They also require a similar active submission in order to work properly: universal terminologies have to be actively articulated to local dialects in order for the terminology to be practical, and for the dialects to be translated and classified (Bowker and Star 1999).

Compared to the procedural standards discussed here, however, it is clear that most terminological standards will have a much less clear presence than these procedural standards. That is to say, in the case of the research protocol or reporting forms discussed here, the health care workers had to pay attention to them and actively orient themselves to them in their work. They were quite visible, for these workers and an external observer alike. Terminological standards, however, may be part and parcel of the categories health care workers already think with, or they may be ingrained in the very words used in the preset text on the forms. In these cases, health care workers use these standards without thinking, and an observer would notice them only if he or she knew where to look for them. Such standards have become part of the infrastructure of these practices (Star and Ruhleder 1996); they have sunk into the background, structuring the work, aligning it with the work of other groups, without anyone paying notice anymore.

This phenomenon can also occur with procedural standards: guidelines can become so ingrained in the routines of health care workers, for example, that these health care workers are not even aware of the fact that they are following a procedural standard. Does this mean, however, that in these cases these standards structure work without the active counter-role for the health care worker that we stated to be so crucial? We would argue that in these cases, what becomes routinized in the actions of health care workers is exactly this position of active submission. In these cases, the health care worker does indeed not reconsider, each and every time, just how far she or he will allow the standard to affect her or him, and vice versa. Yet what becomes routinized is the *outcome* of this negotiation process: the moments where the standard is followed precisely, the moments where shortcuts are taken, the new skills and new activities that the standard require and make possible.

As Schmidt and Werle argued, design and performance standards are likewise coordinating devices as far as they ensure mutual compatibility between individual entities of a system—whether a fax machine's components or the National Institute of Social Insurance's administrative bodies. For these types of standards, this clearly involves a delegation of coordinating activities to the standards (from, in this case, the designers/managers of these systems): in meeting the standards' requirements, a match with external expectations and interchangeability of the constituting components are partially guaranteed.

45. Gomart and Hennion 1999; Gomart 2003.
46. Berg 1997; Star and Strauss 1997.
47. Shapin 1989; Star 1991.

Chapter 3. From Autonomy to Accountability

1. Sanders 1999, 119; Merritt et al. 1997.
2. McIntyre 2001, S338.
3. Timmermans 1999b.
4. Sanders 1999, 121.
5. Tunis et al. 1994b.
6. As discussed in Chapter 6, prescribing drugs off-label refers to the physician's professional prerogative to prescribe drugs for conditions other than the ones the drug was approved for by the U.S. Food and Drug Administration.
7. Freidson 1986, 204.
8. Abbott 1988, 20.
9. Light 1993.
10. Abbott 1988, 102.
11. In this sense, the continuing development of medical guidelines reflects the medicalization of everyday life. But it also explains why not every aspect of life will be medicalized. Claiming entire new jurisdictions might damage an established profession—like medicine—because it runs the risk of weakening the accepted body of knowledge (Abbott 1988). Professional autonomy requires specialized knowledge, not a renaissance sense of expertise.
12. Mulrow 1994; Cochrane Collaboration 1999.
13. ACOG 1997.
14. Ibid., 5.
15. Porter 1997; Berg 1997b. It should be remarked that what scientific exactly *meant*, and *how* exactly this scientific character of medicine could be enhanced, was not a given feature and varied markedly during this episode. Even during the postwar period, not one single definition of scientificness stood uncontested. In fact, the current epidemiological, empiricist definitions of evidence and science are but one possible way one could define the scientific character of medicine, another one being more rooted in biomedical sciences such as physiology and molecular biology (Feinstein 1987).
16. Porter 1997.
17. Becker et al. 1961; Fox 1957, 1980; Light 1979.
18. Benner 1984; Freidson 1970; Dreyfus and Dreyfus 1986.
19. Friedland 1999; Evidence Based Medicine Working Group 1992.

20. Friedland 1999; Evidence Based Medicine Working Group 1992.

21. Paauw 1999.

22. Whether economic considerations should or should not be central to the evidence that medicine should be based upon is a matter of debate within the evidence-based medicine movement. Some argue that such considerations do not belong in this category; others counter that the medical profession can no longer close their eyes to the realities of limited budgets and priority-setting needs (Wynia 1997; Clancy and Kamerow 1996; Eddy 1993).

23. Council 1948. The Hill clinical trial was "first" in the sense that it mobilized a general medical audience to the benefits of clinical trials. Whether it was an historical first remains debated (see Hrobjartsson et al. 1998).

24. Abraham 1995.

25. Matthews 1995, 139.

26. Porter 1995.

27. Whether nursing is an emerging or established profession remains a topic of debate: see Coburn 1988; Beardwood 2000; Furlong and Wilken 1998.

28. This case study is based upon Timmermans et al. 1998. See also Bowker and Star 1999.

29. McCloskey and Bulechek 2000.

30. Brannon 1994.

31. In addition to the fact that nursing research is largely underfunded, one of the limitations of randomized clinical trials is their inadequacy for evaluating interventions. Randomized clinical trials have not been widespread in the evaluation of surgical or nursing interventions: their main application domain has been drug testing. The advantage of canvassing the nursing profession was that it sensitized the emerging profession to the making of the intervention classification system.

32. Lohr et al. 1998.

33. Hess 1998, 17.

34. Smith 2000, S12.

35. Freidson 1986, 204, our emphasis.

36. Mitchell 2000.

37. Woolf et al. 1999, 530.

38. One of the ironies of EBM is that clinical practice guidelines are often evaluated with research that does not conform to the highest level of evidence. Most evaluative studies rely on self-reports and self-assessmentes or on chart reviews. According to one of EBM's founders, besides methodological problems, conceptual weaknesses abound as well (Sackett et al. 2000, 7).

39. Arroll et al. 1995.

40. Christakis and Rivara 1998.

41. Donaldson et al. 1999.

42. Grol et al. 1998.

43. Rhew et al. 1998.

44. Mitchell 2000.

45. Weiss and Wagner 2000.

46. Grilli and Lomas 1994.

47. Wennberg 1999.

48. Eisenberg 1999, 1866; Klazinga 1994.

49. Griffen and Fischer 1997, 31.

50. Jackson and Feder 1998.

51. For a review, see Weingarten 2000. With regard to the standards-upon-standards, Ken Alder has pointed out that such cascades generate more potential detours and problems and are by definition insufficient for the purpose of achieving absolute uniformity or objectivity. He concludes that "the price of standards is eternal vigilance" (Alder 1998, 528).

52. Freidson 1986, 228–229.

53. Abbott 1988, 25.

54. Hughes 1988.

55. ACOG 1997, 6.

56. Armstrong 2002, 1774.

57. Sackett and Rosenberg 1995, 71.

58. Isaacs and Fitzgerald 1999.

59. Tanenbaum 1994.

60. Anonymous quoted in Houtchens et al. 1995, 93.

61. Woolf et al. 1999, 529.

62. Zinberg 1998.

63. Woolf et al. 1996.

64. "Clinical governance is a system through which NHS organizations are accountable for continuously improving the quality of their services and safeguarding high standards of care by creating an environment in which excellence in clinical care will flourish" (Scally and Donaldson 1998, 61).

65. Schlesinger et al. 1997, 106.

66. Wolff and Schlesinger 1998.

67. This is also called "precertification," and it is the most common form of utilization review. Other forms are concurrent review, second opinions, and case management for high-cost patients.

68. Fielding 1990.

69. See Strumwasser et al. 1990. Rosoff (2001, 238) notes that "it is instructive to note that clinical practice guidelines developed from EBM rather than through a professional consensus process differ in this regard from the more traditional Medicare utilization review protocols, which were statutorily required to be based upon 'professionally developed norms of care, diagnosis, and treatment based upon typical patterns of practice.'" He notes that other observers consider the Medicare guidelines more pejoratively only concerned with cost containment and thus have little relevance to quality of care debates. While most commentators would indeed consider utilization review protocols different from clinical practice guidelines, we are here interested in how the tools of evidence-based medicine are used as leverage points in attempts to control costs

by managed care organizations. Also, some observers note that the EBM movement and the utilization review movement are closely intertwined: Medicare
carriers have been "developing clinical guidelines with state medical boards to
support their reimbursement authorization process" (Grogan et al. 1994, 9). See
also Belkin 1997.

70. Schlesinger et al. 1997, 108.
71. Ibid., 115.
72. Levine 1987.
73. Wolff and Schlesinger 1998.
74. Grogan et al. 1994.
75. Greco and Eisenberg 1993.
76. Merritt et al. 1997, 109.
77. Zinberg 1998.
78. ACOG 1996, 92.
79. Doyle 1953.
80. Bickell et al. 1995.
81. Bernstein et al. 1993.
82. Weiss and Wagner 2000.
83. This case study is based upon Rappolt 1997.
84. Rappolt 1997, 982.
85. With the Labour government of Tony Blair, a government white paper on
the National Health Service (NHS) in England outlines a renewed health care
system in which all health organizations will have the statutory duty to seek
continuous and systematic quality improvement through "clinical governance"
(Secretary of State for Health 1997).
86. Light 2000, 206.
87. Millenson 1997.
88. Belkin 1997, 509.
89. Ibid., 524.
90. E.g., Freidson 1989.
91. Ibid., 197.
92. E.g., Saver 1996; Vakil 2001; Rodwin 2001; Belkin 1997.
93. Sonnad and Foreman 1997; Smith 2000.
94. Curry 2000.
95. Rosoff 2001.
96. Federal rules of evidence, rules 401, 402, 403.
97. Jacobson 1997, 74H. Also, see Rosoff 2001 for more detail on the different
legal standards.
98. Rosoff 2001, 328.
99. Matthews 1999, 289.
100. Eisenberg 2001.
101. Rosoff 2001.
102. Hyams et al. 1995.

103. Rosoff 2001, 341.
104. Hyams et al. 1996.
105. Hyams et al. 1995.
106. Rosoff 2001, 344.
107. Griffen and Fischer 1997, 32.
108. Jacobson 1997, H74.
109. Hozer 1990.
110. Eckle and Gausche-Hill 2001.
111. Light and Hughes 2001.
112. Lohr et al. 1998, 5.
113. Tunis et al. 1994.
114. E.g., Bohigian 1988; Kaufman 1993.
115. See overview in Light and Levine 1988 and in Freidson 1989.
116. Light 2000, 207.
117. Light 1993, 36.
118. Smith 2000, S14.
119. Davis and Taylor-Vaisey 1997.
120. Armstrong 2002, 1776.
121. Heffner 2000.
122. Katz 1999.
123. Rolnick, Flores, O'Fallon, and Vanderburg 2000, 35.
124. Savoie, Kazanjian, and Bassett 2000.

Chapter 4. Guidelines, Professionals, and the Production of Objectivity in Insurance Medicine

1. Dodier 1994.
2. Daston and Galison 1992.
3. Knorr-Cetina 1996; Stengers 1997; Berg and Mol 1998.
4. Porter 1995; Alder 1998; Lachmund 1998.
5. Latour 1987a; Shapin and Schaffer 1985.
6. Pasveer 1989; Blume 1992; Howell 1995.
7. See Chapter 2, note 1.
8. Meershoek 1999; Dodier 1994.
9. www.lisv.nl
10. www.ctsv.nl
11. LISV 1997.
12. Porter 1995; Abbott 1988; Freidson 1989.
13. Unless listed otherwise, the quotes in this section derive from the standard that is discussed.
14. Freidson 1989.
15. Meershoek 1999.

16. Horstman 1999.

17. Not all insurance physicians agreed with the specific interpretation of "objective determination" of a claim and the specific position of the client achieved in these guidelines. Within the Netherlands, some insurance physicians argue that objectivity should be interpreted much more narrowly, and that insurance medicine can only truly grow in status and fulfill its legal role when it embraces a strictly biomedical notion of causality and disturbance. The guidelines, thus, should not be seen only as instruments in an ongoing discussion between insurance physicians and their environment: they are similarly part and parcel of an ongoing battle of defining the essence of insurance medicine *within* the profession itself.

18. This apparent contradiction is only partial, because some of the explicit criteria themselves require much interpretation. An important criterion for NLAP, for example, is the "incapacity to function personally or socially." To determine whether this criterion is applicable, the insurance physician again acts fully according to the outlined MDC philosophy.

19. Rothman 1991; Smith 1990.

20. Haraway 1991.

21. All these wordings are derived from actual insurance physician's records. See Berg (1996) for a study of the core role of record-keeping activities in medical work. The phenomenon described here has its historical precedents. One of the core theoretical/political debates during the scientific revolution was exactly *who* counted as a trustworthy witness to a scientific experiment: not poor people, for example, or women (Shapin and Schaffer 1985; Haraway 1997).

22. Porter 1995, 4.

23. Abbott 1988; Löwy 1997.

24. Porter 1995, 8.

25. Woolf et al. 1999; Freidson 1989.

26. According to mechanical rules, cf. Porter 1995, 3–5.

27. Gomart and Hennion 1999.

28. See note 17.

CHAPTER 5. EVIDENCE-BASED MEDICINE AND LEARNING TO DOCTOR

1. For example, Ghali et al. 2000; Green 1999; Kasuya and Sakai 1996; Nony et al. 1999; Welch and Lurie 2000.

2. AAMC 2000.

3. Eisenberg 1999, 1868.

4. Hurwitz 1999, 661.

5. All names of residents are pseudonyms to protect confidentiality and anonymity.

6. Bazarian et al. 1999.

7. Barnett et al. 2000.
8. Norman and Shannon 1998.
9. Potential respondents received a notice about the study from the chief resident. They then contacted the researchers and set up an interview time. Even with the blessing of the attending, it remained difficult and time-consuming to access the residency programs. Chief residents remained protective of the residents' time. We managed to interview 45 percent of the residents in both programs. No one refused the interview after contacting us. The interviews were tape-recorded and lasted about an hour, with a couple interviews lasting up to two and a half hours. All respondents were asked similar questions aimed at generating detailed stories but not necessarily in the same wording and sequence. Wording and sequence depended on the flow of the interview and the responses provided. The interviews were transcribed and went through successive rounds of open, selective, and axial coding (Strauss 1987).

This study is limited in two important ways. First, the use of in-depth interviews limits the understanding of the role of EBM. Because we were interested in how EBM has permeated the trainees' practice we would have preferred to observe residents in their clinical decision making and patient contacts. Unfortunately, because of the above-mentioned access issues, such a study was not feasible. To compensate for our lack of observational data, we probed repeatedly for specific and detailed instances of clinical problem solving. Still, interview data does not allow us to assess with the same precision as observational data how common, for example, computer searches are in the residents' workdays.

A second limitation is our small sample size and our deliberate choice to limit our study to one of the most EBM-saturated medical subdisciplines: pediatrics. The small sample size does not allow us to make fine distinctions along the lines of gender, race, medical subdiscipline, and year of residency—all potentially relevant independent variables. Instead of untenably fragmenting the data and providing speculative interpretations based on one or two residents, we decided to analyze our data on the level of pediatric residents and make distinctions on analytical grounds. This methodological strategy fits in with grounded theory's principle of theoretical sampling: interviewing and analysis is guided by emerging conceptual categories until data saturation is reached (Glaser and Strauss 1967). In this approach, the size of the study matters for the conceptual density of the findings but not necessarily for generalizability across populations.

10. Fox 1957.
11. Bird et al. 2000.
12. Hafferty 2000, 252.
13. Grimes 1995.
14. Bordley et al. 1997, 428.
15. Bazarian et al. 1999, 152.
16. Green 1999, 687, italics in original.
17. See, for example, Fox 2000.
18. Freidson 1994; Hughes 1971 (1945).

19. Siberry and Iannone 2000.

20. Graef 1997.

21. www.aap.org/policy/paramtoc.html

22. www.mdconsult.com

23. Sackett et al. 1996, 71.

24. Atkinson 1984; Fox 1980; Light 1979.

25. Fox 1957.

26. Fox 1980, 2000.

27. Atkinson 1984; Katz 1984; Light 1979.

28. Light 1979.

29. Atkinson 1984, 954.

30. Katz 1984.

31. Only Light and Katz focus their writing on the socialization of residents, but Fox and Atkinson imply that uncertainty and control have relevance for residency training.

32. Fox 2000.

33. Fox 1980, 7.

34. Hardern 1999.

35. Grimes 1995, 453.

36. Evidence Based Medicine Working Group 1992.

37. Sackett et al. 1985.

38. Bosk 1980, 73.

39. Good 1998.

40. See also Anspach 1993; Collins 1985.

41. Latour 1999, 46.

42. Conrad 1988.

43. Evidence Based Medicine Working Group 1992.

44. Sackett et al. 1996.

45. Fox 1957; Haas and Shaffir 1987; Merton et al. 1957.

46. Freidson 1986.

47. See Anspach 1993.

Chapter 6. Standardizing Risk

1. Lewis 2001.

2. Celgene's case was slightly different since it came in under orphan drug status. An orphan drug (i.e., a drug that is aimed at a treatment for a condition with relative few sufferers) has to fulfill less stringent scientific criteria as part of its approval process.

3. Relman 1980.

4. Etminan et al. 1998.

5. Smart and Williams 1997.

6. Garattini 1998.

7. Tallon et al. 2000.

8. U.S. Preventive Services Task Force 1996.

9. Berg et al. 2001.

10. Bowker and Star 1999.

11. Vaughan 1996.

12. Beck 1992.

13. Perrow 1984.

14. Latour 1987; Callon 1986.

15. The full transcripts are available at:
http://www.fda.gov/cder/thalinfo/332t11.rtf
http://www.fda.gov/cder/news/thalinfo/332t12.rtf
http://www.fda.gov/oashi/patrep/nih99.html
http://www.fda.gov/oashi/patrep/nih910.html

16. Matthews 1995.

17. Fine 1972.

18. Connors 1996.

19. Abraham 1995.

20. Krantz 1978.

21. Asbury 1985.

22. Lou Morris, Ph.D., chief, Division of Drug Marketing, Advertising and Communications, CDER, FDA (10 September), 5.

23. A National Library of Medicine bibliography listed 1,495 citations out of more than 4,600 between January 1963 and July 1997 (Patrias et al. 1997).

24. Among the conditions are: skin disorders (prurigo nodularis and photo-dermatitis, leprosy and erythema nodosum leprosum, Behçet's disease, and pyoderma gangrenosum); immunologic and rheumatologic disorders (lupus erythematosus, arthritis, Crohn's disease, and ulcerative colitis); hematologic and oncologic disorders (glioma, prostate cancer, graft versus host disease, Kaposi's sarcoma, and breast cancer); and infectious diseases (tuberculosis, HIV/AIDS and AIDS wasting syndrome, and apthous ulcers).

25. Thalidomide is similar to DES in its potential for benefits and potential for harm. Susan Bell's analysis of the history of the FDA's approval of DES points out that a great deal of medical attention was focused on DES, because of this high-stakes risk-benefit analysis (Bell 1995).

26. Because of the low numbers of thalidomide babies born in the United States, no victims' association exists there. The Canadian association has reached out to the U.S. Thalidomiders and presents itself as their spokesperson.

27. Bruce Williams, vice president, Sales and Marketing, Celgene Corporation (4 September), 78; (10 September), 26–31.

28. The participants did not explain how one "proves" a missed period.

29. Abbott 1988.

30. Cynthia Pearson, National Women's Health Network (9 September), 52.

31. Ibid.

32. Randolph Warren, CEO, Thalidomide Victim's Association of Canada (5 September), 54.

33. Gail Povar, George Washington University School of Medicine (10 September), 18.

34. James Allen, M.D., American Medical Association (9 September), 49.

35. Mark Senak, J.D., AIDS Project Los Angeles (10 September), 22.

36. Gail Povar, George Washington University School of Medicine (10 September), 19.

37. Thomas Bleakley, J.D., Bleakley & McKeen, P.C. (10 September), 57.

38. Gail Povar, George Washington University School of Medicine (10 September), 20.

39. Similarly, Bell found that science helped to preserve medical power in the case of DES approval in 1941 (Bell 1994).

40. Murray Lumpkin, M.D., deputy center director for review management, CDER, FDA (9 September), 75.

41. Lou Morris, chief, Division of Drug Marketing, Advertising, and Communications, Center for Drug Evaluation and Research, FDA (10 September), 8.

42. Mark Senak, J.D., AIDS Project Los Angeles (10 September), 24.

43. Thomas Rea, Celgene Corporation (5 September), 90.

44. Barbara Hill, Division of Dermatological and Dental Drug Products, Center for Drug Evaluation and Research, FDA (9 September), 97.

45. Martin Fishbein, Ph.D., University of Pennsylvania (10 September), 12.

46. Lou Morris, Ph.D., chief, Division of Drug Marketing, Advertising, and Communications, CDER, FDA (10 September) 8.

47. As was widely publicized in the U.S. news media, several health maintenance organizations do not cover contraceptives for women, although they do cover the male impotency drug Viagra.

48. People diagnosed with leprosy were escorted by law officials to Carville, their possessions were burned, and, if they died, their graves would often be marked with assumed names. Carville was basically a total institution modeled after a prison (Goffman 1961; Gussow 1989).

49. Leo Yoder, M.D., American Leprosy Mission (4 September), 44.

50. Mark Senak, J.D., AIDS Project Los Angeles (10 September), 93.

51. Epstein 1996.

52. Ibid., 24.

53. Ibid., 36.

54. Christine Mauck, M.D., M.P.H., Division of Reproductive and Urologic Drug Products, Center for Drug Evaluation and Research, FDA (9 September), 92–93.

55. Cynthia Pearson, National Women's Health Network (9 September), 52.

56. Leo Yoder, M.D., American Leprosy Mission (4 September), 43.

57. Christine Mauck, M.D., M.P.H., Division of Reproductive and Urologic Drug Products, Center for Drug Evaluation and Research, FDA (9 September), 95.

58. Christine Mauck, M.D., M.P.H., Division of Reproductive and Urologic

Drug Products, Center for Drug Evaluation and Research, FDA (9 September), 94.

59. Christine Mauck, M.D., M.P.H., Division of Reproductive and Urologic Drug Products, Center for Drug Evaluation and Research, FDA (9 September), 94.

60. Martin Fishbein, Ph.D., University of Pennsylvania (10 September), 10.

61. There was uncertainty regarding thalidomide's possible effects on sperm. The researchers decided that it was better to take precautions.

62. S.T.E.P.S. information packet for prescribers and patients. The packet contains two brochures published by the Planned Parenthood organization: one about emergency contraception, the other about "your contraceptive choices." The packet notes: "Remember that the only method of birth control that is 100% effective is not having sex at all."

63. Norman Fost, M.D., M.P.H., University of Wisconsin–Madison (9 September), 28.

64. Bruce Williams, Celgene Corporation (10 September), 30.

65. There is a large literature on precedents with similar outcomes. See, for example, Clarke 1998; Franklin 1997; Ginsberg and Rapp 1995; Donchin 1996; Hartouni 1997; Martin 1987.

66. Franklin 1997.

67. "Do we like thalidomide?" Warren asked. "No. The word to us is poison. That's what it is. Skulls, crossbones, poison" (Randolph Warren, CEO, Thalidomide Victim's Association of Canada [5 September], 52).

68. Ibid., 54.

69. Ibid.

70. Implicitly, and sometimes quite explicitly during the meetings, various participants voiced the view that the lives of thalidomide babies were not worth living and that their births should be avoided at all costs. A consumer advocate, for example, noted the family trauma, divorce, and "everything else that goes with it" that disability causes (Susan Cohen, FDA consumer representative [4 September], 154). Others similarly pointed to the drawbacks and negatives of disabled life, even equating it with child abuse, misery, and suffering (Norman Fost, M.D., MPH, University of Wisconsin–Madison [9 September], 63). While most disability advocates fiercely object to such depictions and assumptions of people with disabilities as problem-prone, victimized, and somehow deficient (there exists a broad literature on this topic; see, for example, Morris 1991) the Thalidomiders labeled themselves "victims."

71. Randolph Warren, CEO, Thalidomide Victim's Association of Canada (5 September), 43.

72. Bruce Williams, Celgene Corporation (5 September), 89.

73. Lambert 1996.

74. Phipps 1990.

75. Sitkin and Sutcliffe 1991.

76. William A. Zellmer, MPH, American Society of Health System Pharmacists (9 September), 47.

77. Susan Winckler, American Pharmaceutical Association (10 September), 62.

78. William A. Zellmer, American Society of Health System Pharmacists (9 September), 47.

79. Thomas Bleakley, J.D., Bleakley & McKeen, P.C. (10 September), , 61.

80. Abraham and Sheppard 1998.

81. Epstein 1996; Vogel 1990.

82. Abraham and Sheppard 1998.

83. Jasanoff 1990.

84. The members of the FDA advisory committee were aware that the biggest market for thalidomide consisted of AIDS patients, but because considerably more research existed on the effects of thalidomide on ENL than on other conditions, the application was made for that condition, and assigned to the dermatology section for review.

85. The advisory committee meeting consisted of presentations and discussion about the safety, efficacy, and indication of thalidomide, and a discussion of the distribution system. We do not focus on the presentation of scientific evidence, but note that by all accounts the documentation of thalidomide's safety was insufficient. The FDA's own scientific safety reviewers and the advisory panel rejected the drug's safety claims largely because the historical and experimental trials did not come close to meeting the standards of clinical trials in the 1990s. The efficacy claims were also shaky: one committee member stated that "I have faith that the drug is effective, but scientifically I don't believe the data support that it's effective. . . . If this weren't an orphan drug, it would not have been at this level of a meeting" (Joel Mindel, M.D., director, Neuro-Ophthalmology, Mt. Sinai Hospital, New York [5 September], 66). For an account of the inconclusiveness of scientific data in the controversy of the effectiveness of vitamin C as a therapy against cancer, see Richard 1991.

86. Randolph Warren, CEO, Thalidomide Victim's Association of Canada (9 September), 56.

87. Janet Woodcock, M.D., director, Center for Drug Evaluation and Research, FDA (10 September), 86.

88. Thomas Bleakley, J.D., Bleakley & McKeen, P.C. (10 September), 47.

89. Abraham 1994; Mann 1987.

90. Welsh 1995.

91. Celgene's board includes a former FDA commissioner, Arthur Hull Hayes (http://www.celgene.com).

92. Sunday Times Insight Team 1979.

93. Abraham 1994.

94. Gail Povar, George Washington University School of Medicine (10 September), 16.

95. Iris Long, M.D., ACT UP/New York (10 September), 78.

96. Except for the drugs that are part of a system of mandatory restricted distribution.

97. Steve Thomas, Celgene Corporation (5 September), 129.

98. Forsythe 1996.

99. Akrich 1992, 210.

100. Bowker and Star 1999, 140.

101. Jasanoff 1990.

102. For a similar case where such assumptions were unwarranted, see Rapp 1998.

103. Thomas Bleakley, J.D., Bleakley & McKeen, P.C. (10 September), 50.

104. Janet Woodcock, M.D., director, CDER, FDA (10 September) 86.

105. Bowker 1993; Porter 1995.

106. Cynthia Moore, M.D., Ph.D., Birth Defects and Genetic Disease Branch, Centers for Disease Control and Prevention (4 September), 146.

107. Vaughan 1996.

108. Fujimura 1987.

Epilogue

1. Committee on Quality of Health Care in America 2000.

2. See, for example, Latham 2001; Sox and Woloshin 2000.

3. Committee on Quality of Health Care in America 2000, 44–53.

4. Ibid., 28–30.

5. Chassin et al. 1998. The Urgent Need to Improve Health Care Quality. *Journal of the American Medical Association* 280: 1000–1005. Quoted in ibid., 23–24.

6. Measuring hemoglobin A1c is a means to check whether the glucose level of the patient is within the optimal range.

7. Wiener 2000.

8. Ibid., 133, 192.

9. S. Skillihorn (1980). *Quality and Accountability: A New Era in American Hospitals.* San Francisco: Editorial Consultants, 32. In Wiener (2000, 133).

10. Wiener seems torn by these issues. In her book, she partially embraces the first committee's report when she states that errors are a huge problem in current medical care. In her analysis of the weaknesses of the accountability quest, she stresses that errors are usually downplayed and acted upon defensively (204–211). In this way, while overlooking how a focus on errors has become one of the core drivers of the accountability movement, she suddenly—and without explanation—sides with the analysis of current medicine she criticizes in the rest of her book.

11. Committee on Quality of Health Care in America 2000, 53.

12. While critics of "technoscience" often blame quality protagonists and the likes for holding on to these simplifications, these protagonists themselves are often much smarter than their critics would like to believe. See, for example, Latour 1996; Berg et al. 2001.

13. Again, we are fully aware of the fact that we can deconstruct all of these statements—as if full articulation is possible, or as if information is something that can be simply transmitted over time and place. Simply deconstructing problems, however, does not make them go away.

14. Wiener 2000, 96.

15. Committee on Quality of Health Care in America 2001, 145.

16. Lawrence Weed is quoted without reference. Weed would probably want to remedy his eloquent diagnosis with a highly elaborate decision support system, which will apply this medical knowledge to any patient's problem for the doctor (cf. Weed 1985). See Berg 1997b for a critique of such approaches.

17. For a beautiful illustration of the latter, see Hutchins 1995.

18. See Berg 1997b for a detailed analysis.

19. Committee on Quality of Health Care in America 2001, 181–206.

20. Which is not to say, of course, that these drives may not be subtly rechanneled in the process.

21. Berwick 1998a.

22. McGlynn 1998; Millenson 1997.

23. The report is less outspoken about this distinction than, for example, Berwick is. Yet the preference for this approach is clearly present. See pp. 135–137.

24. Millenson 1997. The report glosses over these issues. It talks little about the current rush for accountability measures in the United States. It does mention the manifold problems plaguing "quality measurement for external accountability" (102–103), but it mainly emphasizes measurement in the context of feedback and process improvement.

25. Berwick 1998b.

26. This expression is from Abbott (1988b).

27. In using the term *redesign*, we do not imply that changing an organization is a simple reengineering exercise. Even if one realizes that organizational change comes erratically, in small steps that can never be fully planned, it remains important to try to set aims that are both realistic and ambitious. Put more positively, terms like *redesign* are not anathema to sociologically sensitive analyses of work (Suchman 1987; Brown and Duguid 2000). Rather, proper redesign can take place only when building upon the latter's insights.

28. Collen 1995.

29. Thanks to Mario Stefanelli for this phrasing.

30. Massaro 1993, 22.

31. McDonald et al. 1984; van der Lei et al. 1993.

32. Schmidt and Bannon 1992.

33. Winthereik in press.

34. Berg and Toussaint in press.
35. Bowker and Star 1999.
36. Lundberg and Hanseth 2001; Ellingsen and Monteiro forthcoming.
37. Groth 1999.
38. Berg 1997b; Forsythe 2001; Brown and Duguid 2000.
39. Brown and Duguid 2000.
40. Hartswood et al. 2000.
41. There are many different names for this multifaceted movement; we do not intend to pinpoint one specific branch by using this name.

Bibliography

AAMC. 2000. *A Century of Reform: Medical Education's Quiet Revolution to Meet America's Health Care Needs*. Washington, DC: American Association of Medical Colleges.

Abbott, A. 1988. *The System of Professions*. Chicago: University of Chicago Press.

Abraham, J. 1994. Distributing the Benefit of the Doubt: Scientists, Regulators, and Drug Safety. *Science, Technology, and Human Values* 19: 493–522.

———. 1995. *Science, Politics and the Pharmaceutical Industry: Controversy and Bias in Drug Regulation*. London: UCL Press.

Abraham, J., and J. Sheppard. 1998. International Comparative Analysis and Explanation in Medical Sociology: Demystifying the Halcion Anomaly. *Sociology* 32: 29–51.

ACOG. 1996. Laparoscopically Assisted Vaginal Hysterectomy. *International Journal of Gynecology and Obstetrics* 53: 91–92.

———. 1997. Routine Ultrasound in Low-Risk Pregnancy. *Practice Patterns* 1–5.

Akrich, M. 1992. The De-Scription of Technical Objects. In *Shaping Technology/Building Society: Studies in Sociotechnical Change*, edited by W. Bijker and J. Law, 205–224. Cambridge, MA: MIT Press.

Alder, K. 1998. Making Things the Same: Representation, Tolerance and the End of the Ancien Regime in France. *Social Studies of Science* 28: 499–545.

American Heart Association. 1990. *Textbook of Advanced Cardiac Life Support*. Dallas: American Heart Association.

Anonymous. 1904. Hospital "Bedside Notes" Not Admissible in Evidence. *Journal of the American Medical Association* 43: 380.

Anonymous. 1912. The Care of Hospital Records. *The Lancet* 805.

Anonymous. 1914. Standardization in Hospital Records. *Boston Medical and Surgical Journal* 170: 63.

Anonymous. 1916. Improvement in Medical Statistics. *Journal of the American Medical Association* 66: 634.

Anonymous. 1924. Onderling vergelijkbare boekhouding in de ziekenhuizen. *Het Ziekenhuis* 15: 123–127.

Anonymous. 1929a. Boekbespreking "Rationalisierung klinischer betriebe, von Dr. Werner Nissel." *Het Ziekenhuiswezen* 2: 280.

Anonymous. 1929b. Developing the Record Department in the Small Hospital. *Modern Hospital* 32: 88.

Anonymous. 1929c. Tube System Facilitates Record Service. *Modern Hospital* 33: 68.

Anonymous. 1933. Admissibility of Hospital Records and Charts as Evidence. *Modern Hospital* 40: 82.

Anspach, R. 1993. *Deciding Who Lives: Fateful Choices in the Intensive Care Nursery.* Berkeley: University of California Press.

Armstrong, D. 2002. Clinical Autonomy, Individual and Collective: The Problem of Changing Doctors' Behaviour. *Social Science and Medicine* 55(10): 1771–1779.

Aronowitz, R. A. 1998. *Making Sense of Illness.* Cambridge: Cambridge University Press.

Arroll, B., S. Jenkins, D. North, and R. Kearns. 1995. Management of Hypertension and the Core Services Guidelines: Results from Interviews with 100 Auckland General Practitioners. *New Zealand Medical Journal* 108: 55–57.

Asbury, C. H. 1985. *Orphan Drugs: Medical versus Market Value.* Lexington, MA: Lexington Books.

Atkinson, P. 1984. Training for Certainty. *Social Science and Medicine* 19: 949–956.

Atwater, E. C. 1989. Women, Surgeons, and Worthy Enterprise: The General Hospital Comes to Upper New York State. In *The American General Hospital,* edited by D. E. Long and J. L. Golden, 40–66. Ithaca and London: Cornell University Press.

Auchincloss, H. 1989 (1926). Unit History System. In *Technology and American Practice 1880–1930,* edited by J. D. Howell, 306–316. New York and London: Garland Publishing.

Bachmeyer, A. C. 1922a. Administrative Records for the Hospital. *Modern Hospital* 19: 39–40.

———. 1922b. Professional Records for the Hospital. *Modern Hospital* 19: 227–228.

Barnett, S. H., S., Kaiser, K. L. Morgan, J. Sullivant, A. Sie, D. Rose, M. Ricota, L. Smith, C. Schechter, M. Miller, and A. Stagnard-Green. 2000. An Integrated Program for Evidence-Based Medicine in Medical School. *Mount Sinai Journal of Medicine* 67: 163–168.

Barrett, R. J. 1988. Clinical Writing and the Documentary Construction of Schizophrenia. *Culture, Medicine and Psychiatry* 12: 265–299.

Bazarian, J. J., C. O. Davis, L. L. Spillane, H. Blumstein, and S. M. Schneider. 1999. Teaching Emergency Medicine Residents Evidence-Based Critical Appraisal Skills: A Controlled Trial. *Annals of Emergency Medicine* 34: 148–154.

Beardwood, B. 2000. The Loosening of Professional Boundaries and Restructuring: The Implications for Nursing and Medicine in Ontario, Canada. *Law and Policy* 21: 315–343.

Beck, U. 1992. *Risk Society: Towards a New Modernity.* London and Newbury Park, CA: Sage Publications.

Becker, H. S., B. Geer, E. C. Hughes, and A. L. Strauss. 1961. *Boys in White.* Chicago: University of Chicago Press.

Becker, L. B. 1993. Methodology in Cardiac Arrest Research Symposium. *Annals of Emergency Medicine* 22: 1–3.

Belkin, G. S. 1997. Sense and Finding Power in the "Managed" Medical Marketplace. *Journal of Health Politics, Policy and Law* 22: 509–532.

Bell, S. E. 1994. From Local to Global: Resolving Uncertainty About the Safety of DES in Menopause. *Research in the Sociology of Health Care* 11: 41–56.

———. 1995. Gendered Medical Science: Producing a Drug for Women. *Feminist Studies* 21: 469–500.

Beniger, J. R. 1986. *The Control Revolution*. Cambridge, MA: Harvard University Press.

Benner, P. 1984. *From Novice to Expert: Excellence and Power in Clinical Nursing Practice*. Menlo Park, CA: Addison-Wesley Publishing Company.

Berg, M. 1996. Practices of Reading and Writing: The Constitutive Role of the Patient Record in Medical Work. *Sociology of Health and Illness* 18: 499–524.

———. 1997a. Of Forms, Containers and the Electronic Medical Record: Some Tools for a Sociology of the Formal. *Science, Technology and Human Values* 22: 403–433.

———. 1997b. *Rationalizing Medical Work: Decision Support Techniques and Medical Practices*. Cambridge, MA: MIT Press.

Berg, M., and P. Harterink. in press. Embodying the Patient: Records and Bodies in Early 20th Century US Medical Practice. *Body and Society*.

Berg, M., R. H. J. t. Meulen, and M. v. d. Burg. 2001. Guidelines for Appropriate Care: The Importance of Empirical Normative Analysis. *Health Care Analysis* 9: 77–99.

Berg, M., and A. Mol, eds. 1998. *Differences in Medicine: Unraveling Practices, Techniques and Bodies*. Durham: Duke University Press.

Berg, M., and P. Toussaint. In press. The Mantra of Modelling and the Forgotten Powers of Paper: A Sociotechnical View on the Development of Process-Oriented ICT in Health Care. *International Journal of Medical Informatics*.

Berkwitz, M. 1998. From Practice to Medicine: The Case for Criticism in an Age of Evidence. *Social Science and Medicine* 47: 1539–1545.

Bernstein, S. J., E. A. McGlynn, A. L. Siu, C. P. Roth, M. J. Sherwood, J. W. Keesey, J. Kosecoff, N. R. Hicks, and R. M. Brook. 1993. The Appropriateness of Hysterectomy: A Comparison of Care in Seven Health Plans. *Journal of the American Medical Association* 269: 2398–2402.

Berwick, D. M. 1998a. Crossing the Boundary: Changing Mental Models in the Service of Improvement. *International Journal of Quality Health Care* 10: 435–441.

———. 1998b. Developing and Testing Changes in Delivery of Care. *Annals of Internal Medicine* 128: 651–656.

Bickell, N. A., J. Earp, A. T. Evans, and S. J. Bernstein. 1995. A Matter of Opinion about Hysterectomies: Experts' and Practicing Community Gynecologists' Ratings of Appropriateness. *American Journal of Public Health* 85: 1125–1128.

Bijker, W. E., and J. Law, eds. 1992. *Shaping Technology—Building Society. Studies in Sociotechnical Change*. Cambridge, MA: MIT Press.

Bird, C. E., P. Conrad, and A. M. Fremont. 2000. *Handbook of Medical Sociology.* Upper-Saddle River, NJ: Prentice-Hall.

Blume, S. S. 1992. *Insight and Industry: On the Dynamics of Technological Change in Medicine.* Cambridge, MA: MIT Press.

Bohigian, G. M. 1988. The Golden Age of Medicine: 1966–1980. *Modern Medicine* 85: 71–74.

Bordley, D. R., M. Fagan, and D. Theige. 1997. Evidence-Based Medicine: A Powerful Educational Tool for Clerkship Education. *American Journal of Medicine* 102: 427–432.

Bosk, C. L. 1980. Occupational Rituals in Patient Management. *New England Journal of Medicine* 303: 71–76.

Bottomley, J. T. 1918. Hospital Standardization—Its Meaning. *Boston Medical and Surgical Journal* 179: 219–223.

Bowker, G. 1993. How to Be Universal: Some Cybernetic Strategies, 1943–70. *Social Studies of Science* 23: 107–127.

Bowker, G. C., and S. L. Star. 1999. *Sorting Things Out.* Cambridge, MA: MIT Press.

Brannon, R. L. 1994. Professionalization and Work Intensification. *Work and Occupations* 21: 157–178.

Brook, R. 1989. Practice Guidelines and Practicing Medicine: Are They Compatible? *Journal of the American Medical Association* 262: 3027–3030.

Brotherhood, J. S. 1913. Hospital Clinical Records. *Journal of the American Medical Association* 60: 1205–1209.

Brough, R. N. 1935. An Important Task Lies with the Record Librarian. *Modern Hospital* 44: 63–64.

Brown, J. S., and P. Duguid. 2000. *The Social Life of Information.* Cambridge, MA: Harvard Business School Press.

Brunsson, N., and B. Jacobsson. 2000. *A World of Standards.* Oxford: Oxford University Press.

Bugbee, G. P. 1932. How Mechanical Aids Facilitate Record Keeping. *Modern Hospital* 38: 144–152.

———. 1935. Simplifying Admitting Records. *Modern Hospital* 45: 41.

Button, G., and R. H. R. Harper. 1993. Taking the Organisation into Accounts. In *Technology in Working Order: Studies of Work, Interaction, and Technology,* edited by G. Button, 98–107. London: Routledge.

Callon, M. 1986. Some Elements of a Sociology of Translation: Domestication of the Scallops and the Fishermen of St Brieuc Bay. In *Power, Action, and Belief: A New Sociology of Knowledge?* edited by J. Law. London: Routledge.

———. 1987. Society in the Making: The Study of Technology as a Tool for Sociological Analysis. In *The Social Construction of Technological Systems,* edited by W. E. Bijker, T. P. Hughes, and T. Pinch, 83–103. Cambridge, MA: MIT Press.

———. 1991. Techno-economic Networks and Irreversibility. In *A Sociology of Monsters: Essays on Power, Technology and Domination,* edited by J. Law, 132–161. London: Routledge.

Cartwright, L. 1995. *Screening the Body: Tracing Medicine's Visual Culture.* Minneapolis: University of Minnesota Press.

Chandler, A. J. 1977. *The Visible Hand: The Managerial Revolution in Business Management.* Cambridge, MA: Harvard University Press.

Charlton, B. G. 1997a. Book Review: Evidence-Based Medicine—How to Practice and Teach EBM. *Journal of Evaluation in Clinical Practice* 3: 169–172.

———. 1997b. Restoring the Balance: Evidence-Based Medicine Put in its Place. *Journal of Evaluation in Clinical Practice* 3: 97–98.

Christakis, D. A., and F. P. Rivara. 1998. Pediatricians' Awareness of and Attitudes about Four Clinical Practice Guidelines. *Pediatrics* 101: 825–830.

Clancy, C. M., and D. B. Kamerow. 1996. Evidence-Based Medicine Meets Cost-Effectiveness Analysis. *Journal of the American Medical Association* 276: 329–330.

Clapesettle, H. 1954. *The Doctors Mayo.* Minneapolis: University of Minnesota Press.

Clarke, A. 1998. *Disciplining Reproduction: Modernity, American Life Sciences, and "The Problems of Sex."* Berkeley: University of California Press.

Coburn, D. 1988. The Development of Canadian Nursing: Professionalization and Proletarization. *International Journal of Health Services* 18: 437–456.

Cochrane Collaboration. 1999. *The Cochrane Library, Update Software, Issue 4.* Oxford, UK: Update Software.

Codman, E. A., W. W. Chipman, J. G. Clark, A. G. Kanaval, and M. J. Mayo. 1914. Report of the Committee on the Standardization of Hospitals. *Boston Medical and Surgical Journal* 170: 71–73.

Coles, J. V. 1949. *Standards and Labels for Consumer Goods.* New York: The Ronald Press Company.

Collen, M. E. 1995. *A History of Medical Informatics in the United States, 1950 to 1990.* Indianapolis: American Medical Informatics Association.

Collins, H. 1985. *Changing Order: Replication and Induction in Scientific Practice.* London: Sage.

Commissie in zake medische statistiek. 1916. Jaarverslag. *Nederlandsch Tijdschrift voor Geneeskunde* 16: 1661–1675.

Committee on Quality of Health Care in America. 2000. *To Err is Human: Building a Safer Health System.* Washington, DC: National Academy Press.

———. 2001. *Crossing the Quality Chasm: A New Health System for the 21st Century.* Washington, DC: National Academy Press.

Connors, T. 1996. Anticancer Drug Development: The Way Forward. *Oncologist* 1: 180–181.

Conrad, P. 1988. Learning to Doctor: Reflections on Recent Accounts of the Medical School Years. *Journal of Health and Social Behavior* 29: 323–332.

Cook, J. E. 1927. How We Facilitate Record Keeping. *Modern Hospital* 24: 69–72.

Council, M. R. 1948. Streptomycin Treatment of Pulmonary Tuberculosis. *British Medical Journal* 769–782.

Craig, B. L. 1989–90. Hospital Records and Record-Keeping, c. 1850–c. 1950. Part I: The Development of Records in Hospitals. *Archivaria* 29: 57–80.

———. 1990. Hospital Records and Record-Keeping, c. 1850–c. 1950. Part II: The Development of Record-Keeping in Hospitals. *Archivaria* 30: 21–38.

Cummins, R. O., J. P. Ornato, W. H. Thies, and P. E. Pepe. 1991. Improving Survival from Sudden Cardiac Arrest: The "Chain of Survival" Concept. *Circulation* 83: 1832–1847.

Curry, S. J. 2000. Organizational Interventions to Encourage Guideline Implementation. *Chest* 118: 40S–46S.

Daston, L., and P. Galison. 1992. The Image of Objectivity. *Representations* 40: 81–129.

Davis, D. A., and A. Taylor-Vaisey. 1997. Translating Guidelines into Practice: A Systematic Review of Theoretical Concepts, Practical Experience, and Research Evidence in the Adoption of Clinical Practice Guidelines. *Canadian Medical Association Journal* 157: 408–416.

Davis, M. M. 1920. New York Dispensaries; Book and Record Keeping. *Modern Hospital* 15: 131–134.

Dick, R. S., E. B. Steen, and D. E. Detmer, eds. 1997. *The Computer-Based Patient Record: An Essential Technology for Health Care.* Washington, DC: National Academy Press.

Dickersin, K., and E. Manheimer. 1998. The Cochrane Collaboration: Evaluation of Health Care and Services Using Systematic Reviews of the Results of Randomized Controlled Trials. *Clinical Obstetrics and Gynecology* 41: 315–331.

Doane, J. C. 1931. Why Hospital Surgical Practice Should Be Standardized. *Modern Hospital* 37: 89–91.

Dodier, N. 1994. Expert Medical Decisions in Occupational Medicine: A Sociological Analysis of Medical Judgement. *Sociology of Health and Illness* 16: 489–514.

Donaldson, J. H., J. H. Hayes, A. G. Barton, D. Howel, and M. Hawthorne. 1999. Impact of Clinical Practice Guidelines on Clinicians' Behaviour: Tonsillectomy in Children. *Journal of Otolaryngology* 28: 24–30.

Donchin, A. 1996. Feminist Critiques of New Fertility Technologies: Implications for Social Policy. *Journal of Medicine and Philosophy* 21: 475–498.

Doyle, J. C. 1953. Unneccessary Hysterectomies: Study of 6248 Operations in Thirty-Five Hospitals during 1948. *Journal of the American Medical Association* 151: 360–365.

Dreyfus, H., and S. E. Dreyfus. 1986. *Mind over Machine: The Power of Human Intuition and Expertise in the Era of the Computer.* Oxford: Blackwell.

Drury, H. B. W. 1922. *Scientific Management: A History and Criticism.* New York: Columbia University Press.

Eckle, N., and M. Gausche-Hill. 2001. Follow New Pediatric Guidelines or Risk Liability. *Hospital Case Management* 9: 135–138.

Eddy, D. M. 1993. Three Battles to Watch in the 1990s. *Journal of the American Medical Association* 270: 520–526.

Eisenberg, J. M. 1999. Ten Lessons for Evidence-Based Technology Assessment. *Journal of the American Medical Association* 282: 1865–1869.

————. 2001. What Does Evidence Mean? Can the Law and Medicine Be Reconciled? *Journal of Health Politics, Policy and Law* 26: 369–381.

Eisenberg, M. S., R. O. Cummins, S. Damon, M. P. Larsen, and T. R. Hearne. 1990a. Survival Rates from Out-of-Hospital Cardiac Arrest: Recommendations for Uniform Definitions and Data to Report. *Annals of Emergency Medicine* 19: 1249–1259.

Eisenberg, M. S., B. T. Horwood, R. O. Cummins, R. Reynolds-Haertle, and T. R. Hearne. 1990b. Cardiac Arrest and Resuscitation: A Tale of 29 Cities. *Annals of Emergency Medicine* 19: 179–186.

Ellingsen, G., and E. Monteiro. Forthcoming. A Patchwork Planet: Integration and Cooperation in Hospitals. *Computer Supported Cooperative Work*

Epstein, S. 1996. *Impure Science: AIDS, Activism, and the Politics of Knowledge.* Berkeley: University of California Press.

————. in press. Bodily Differences and Collective Identities: Representation, Generalizability, and the Politics of Gender and Race in Biomedical Research in the United States. In *Bodies on Trial: Performances and Politics in Medicine and Biology,* edited by M. Akrich and M. Berg. Durham: Duke University Press.

Etminan, M., J. M. Wright, and B. C. Carleton. 1998. Evidence-Based Pharmacotherapy: Review of Basic Concepts and Applications in Clinical Practice. *Annals of Pharmacotherapy* 32: 1193–2000.

Evidence Based Medicine Working Group. 1992. Evidence-Based Medicine: A New Approach to Teaching the Practice of Medicine. *Journal of the American Medical Association* 268: 2420–2425.

Feinstein, A. R. 1987. The Intellectual Crisis in Clinical Science: Medaled Models and Muddled Mettle. *Perspectives in Biology and Medicine* 30: 215–230.

Field, M. J., and K. N. Lohr, eds. 1990. *Clinical Practice Guidelines: Directions for a New Program.* Washington, DC: National Academy Press.

Fielding, S. L. 1990. Physician Reactions to Malpractice Suits and Cost Containment in Massachusetts. *Work and Occupations* 17: 302–319.

Fine, R. A. 1972. *The Great Drug Deception.* New York: Stern and Day.

Forsythe, D. E. 1996. New Bottles, Old Wine: Hidden Cultural Assumptions in a Computerized Explanation System for Migraine Sufferers. *Medical Anthropology Quarterly* 10: 551–574.

————. 2001. *Studying Those Who Study Us: An Anthropologist in the World of Artificial Intelligence.* Stanford: Stanford University Press.

Foucault, M. 1973. *The Birth of the Clinic: An Archaeology of Perception.* New York: Vintage Books.

Fox, R. C. 1957. Training for Uncertainty. In *The Student Physician,* edited by R. K. Merton, G. Reader, and P. L. Kendall. Cambridge, MA: Harvard University Press.

————. 1980. The Evolution of Medical Uncertainty. *Milbank Memorial Fund Quarterly* 58: 1–49.

————. 2000. Medical Uncertainty Revisited. In *The Handbook of Social Studies in Health and Medicine,* edited by G. L. Albrecht, R. Fitzpatrick, and S. C. Scrimshaw, 409–425. London: Sage Publications.

Franklin, S. 1997. *Embodied Progress: A Cultural Account of Assisted Conception.* London and New York: Routledge.

Freeman, A. C., and K. Sweeney. 2001. Why General Practitioners Do Not Implement Evidence: Qualitative Study. *British Medical Journal* 323: 1100.

Freidson, E. 1970. *Profession of Medicine: A Study of the Sociology of Applied Knowledge.* Chicago: University of Chicago Press.

————. 1986. *Professional Powers: A Study of the Institutionalization of Formal Knowledge.* Chicago: Chicago University Press.

————. 1994. *Professionalism Reborn: Theory, Prophecy, and Policy.* Chicago: University of Chicago Press.

————, ed. 1989. *Medical Work in America: Essays on Health Care.* New Haven: Yale University Press.

Friedland, D. J. 1999. *Evidence Based Medicine: A Framework for Clinical Practice.* Stamford, CT: Appleton & Lange.

Fujimura, J. 1987. Constructing "Do-able" Problems in Cancer Research: Articulating Alignment. *Social Studies of Science* 16: 257–293.

Furlong, B., and M. Wilken. 1998. Managed Care and the Nursing Profession. *Research in the Sociology of Health Care* 15: 173–185.

Garattini, S. 1998. The Drug Market in Four European Countries. *Pharmacoeconomics* 14: 69–79.

Garfinkel, H. 1967. *Studies in Ethnomethodology.* Englewood Cliffs, NJ: Prentice-Hall.

Gasser, L. 1986. The Integration of Computing and Routine Work. *ACM Transactions on Office Information Systems* 4: 205–225.

Genevieve Morse, M. 1934. *Hospital Case Records and the Record Librarian.* Chicago: Physicians' Record Co.

Geyman, J. P. 1999. POEMs as a Paradigm Shift in Teaching, Learning and Clinical Practice. *Journal of Family Practice* 48: 343–344.

Ghali, W. A., R. Saitz, A. H. Eskew, M. Gupta, H. Quan, and W. Y. Hershhow. 2000. Successful Teaching in Evidence-Based Medicine. *Medical Education* 34(1): 18–22.

Ginsberg, F., and R. Rapp, eds. 1995. *Conceiving the New World Order: The Global Stratification of Reproduction.* Berkeley: University of California Press.

Ginsburg, W. 1998. Prepare to Be Shocked: The Evolving Standard of Care in Treating Sudden Cardiac Arrest. *American Journal of Emergency Medicine* 16: 315–319.

Glaser, B., and A. Strauss. 1967. *The Discovery of Grounded Theory.* New York: Aldine de Gruyter.

Goffman, E. 1961. *Asylums.* New York: Doubleday.

Gomart, E. 2003 (in press). For a Eulogy of Methadone. *Body and Society.*

————. 2002. Towards Generous Constraint: Freedom and Coercion in a French Addiction Treatment. *Sociology of Health and Illness* 24: 517–550.

Gomart, E., and A. Hennion. 1999. A Sociology of Attachment: Music Amateurs, Drug Users. In *Actor Network Theory and After*, edited by J. Law and J. Hassard, 220–247. Oxford: Blackwell.

Good, M.-J. D. 1998. *American Medicine: The Quest for Competence*. Berkeley: University of California Press.

Graef, J. W. 1997. *Manual of Pediatric Therapeutics*. Philadelphia: Lippincott Raven.

Graham, L. 1998. *Managing on Her Own: Dr. Lilian Gilbreth and Women's Work in the Interwar Era*. Norcross, GA: Engineering and Management Press.

Greco, P. J., and J. M. Eisenberg. 1993. Changing Physicians' Practices. *New England Journal of Medicine* 329: 1271–1274.

Green, J., and N. Britten. 1998. Qualitative Research and Evidence Based Medicine. *British Medical Journal* 316: 1230–1232.

Green, M. L. 1999. Graduate Medical Education Training in Clinical Epidemiology, Critical Appraisal and Evidence-Based Medicine: A Critical Review of Curricula. *Academic Medicine* 74: 686–694.

Griffen, D. F., and J. E. Fischer. 1997. Practice Guidelines and Liability Implications. *Bulletin of the American College of Surgeons* 82: 29–33.

Grilli, R., and J. Lomas. 1994. Evaluating the Relationship between Compliance Rate and the Subject of a Practice Guideline. *Medical Care* 32: 202–213.

Grimes, D. A. 1995. Introducing Evidence-Based Medicine into a Department of Obstetrics and Gynecology. *Obstetrics and Gynecology* 86: 451–457.

Grindley, P. 1995. *Standards Strategy and Policy: Cases and Stories*. Oxford: Oxford University Press.

Grogan, C., R. D. Feldman, J. A. Nyman, and J. Shapiro. 1994. How Will We Use Clinical Guidelines? The Experience of Medicare Carriers. *Journal of Health Politics, Policy, and the Law* 19: 7–26.

Grol, R., J. Dalhuijsen, S. Thomas, C. in 't Veld, G. Rutten, and H. Mokkink. 1998. Attributes of Clinical Guidelines That Influence use of Guidelines in General Practice: Observational Study. *British Medical Journal* 317: 858–861.

Groth, L. 1999. *Future Organizational Design: The Scope for the IT-based Enterprise*. Chichester: Wiley.

Gussow, Z. 1989. *Leprosy, Racism, and Public Health*. Boulder, CO: Westview Press.

Haas, J., and W. Shaffir. 1987. *Becoming Doctors: The Adoption of a Cloak of Competence*. Greenwich, CT: JAI Press.

Hacking, I. 1998. *Mad Travelers: Reflections on the Reality of Transient Mental Illnesses*. Charlottesville and London: University Press of Virginia.

———. 1999. *The Social Construction of What?* Cambridge, MA: Harvard University Press.

Hafferty, F. 2000. Reconfiguring the Sociology of Medical Education: Emerging Topics and Pressing Issues. In *Handbook of Medical Sociology*, edited by C. E. Bird, P. E. Conrad, and A. M. Fremont, 238–257. Upper Saddle River, NJ: Prentice-Hall.

Hanseth, O., E. Monteiro, and M. Hatling. 1996. Developing Information Infrastructure: The Tension between Standardization and Flexibility. *Science, Technology and Human Values* 21: 407–426.

Haraway, D. J. 1991. *Simians, Cyborgs, and Women: The Reinvention of Nature.* New York: Routledge.

———. 1994. A Game of Cat's Cradle: Science Studies, Feminist Theory, Cultural Studies. *Configurations* 1: 59–71.

———. 1997. *Modest_Witness@Second_Millenium_FemaleMan© Meets_ OncoMouse™.* New York: Routledge.

Hardern, R. D. 1999. Teaching and Learning Evidence Based Medicine Skills in Accident and Emergency Medicine. *Journal of Accidents and Emergency Medicine* 16: 126–129.

Hartouni, V. 1997. *Cultural Conceptions: On Reproductive Technologies and the Remaking of Life.* Minneapolis: University of Minnesota Press.

Hartswood, M., R. Procter, M. Rouncefield, and M. Slack. Forthcoming. Making a Case in Medical Work: Implications for the Electronic Medical Record. *Computer Supported Cooperative Work.*

Heffner, J. E. 2000. The Overarching Challenge. *Chest* 118: S1–S3.

Hess, D. 1998. *Can Bacteria Cause Cancer? Alternative Medicine Confronts Big Science.* New York: New York University Press.

Hogle, L. F. 1995. Standardization across Non-standard Domains: The Case of Organ Procurement. In *Constructivist Perspectives on Medical Practices: Medical Practices and Science and Technology Studies. Special Issue of Science, Technology and Human Values,* edited by M. Casper, and M. Berg, 482–500.

Horstman, K. 2000. Technology and the Management of Trust in Insurance Medicine. *Theoretical Medicine and Bioethics* 21(1): 39–61.

Houtchens, B. A., A. Allen, T. P. Clemmer, D. A. Lindberg, and S. Petersem. 1995. Telemedicine Protocols and Standards: Development and Implementation. *Journal of Medical Systems* 19: 93–119.

Howell, J. D. 1989. Machines and Medicine: Technology Transforms the American Hospital. In *The American General Hospital,* edited by D. E. Long and J. Golden, 109–134. Ithaca and London: Cornell University Press.

———. 1995. *Technology in the Hospital: Transforming Patient Care in the Early Twentieth Century.* Baltimore: Johns Hopkins University Press.

Hozer, J. F. 1990. The Advent of Clinical Standards for Professional Liability. *Quality Review Bulletin* 16: 71–79.

Hrobjartsson, A., P. C. Gotzsche, and C. Gluud. 1998. The Controlled Clinical Trial Turns 100 Years: Fibiger's Trial of Serum Treatment of Diphteria. *British Medical Journal* 317: 1243–1245.

Huffman, E. K., and E. Price. 1972. *Medical Record Management.* 6th ed. Berwyn, IL: Physicians' Record Company.

Hughes, A. M. 1932. A Small Hospital Superintendent Explains Her Record System. *Modern Hospital* 38: 95–97.

Hughes, D. 1988. When Nurse Knows Best: Some Observations of Nurse/ Doctor Interaction in a Casualty Department. *Sociology of Health and Illness* 10: 1–22.

Hughes, E. 1971 (1945). *The Sociological Eye: Selected Papers*. Chicago: Aldine-Atherton.

Hurwitz, B. 1999. Legal and Political Considerations of Clinical Practice Guidelines. *British Medical Journal* 318: 661–664.

Hutchins, E. 1995. *Cognition in the Wild*. Cambridge, MA: MIT Press.

Hyams, A. L., J. A. Brandenburg, S. R. Lipsitz, D. W. Shapiro, and T. A. Brennan. 1995. Practice Guidelines and Malpractice Litigation: A Two-Way Street. *Annals of Internal Medicine* 122: 450–455.

Hyams, A. L., D. W. Shapiro, and T. A. Brennan. 1996. Medical Practice Guidelines in Malpractice Litigation: An Early Retrospective. *Journal of Health Politics, Policy, and Law* 21: 289–312.

Ingelfinger, F. J. 1973. Algorithms, Anyone? *New England Journal of Medicine* 288: 847–848.

Isaacs, D., and D. Fitzgerald. 1999. Seven Alternatives to Evidence Based Medicine. *British Medical Journal* 319: 1618.

Jackson, R., and G. Feder. 1998. Guidelines for Clinical Guidelines. *British Medical Journal* 317: 427–428.

Jacobson, P. D. 1997. Legal and Policy Considerations in Using Clinical Practice Guidelines. *American Journal of Cardiology* 80: H74–H79.

Jasanoff, S. 1990. *The Fifth Branch: Science Advisors as Policymakers*. Cambridge, MA: Harvard University Press.

Kasuya, R. T., and D. H. Sakai. 1996. An Evidence-Based Medicine Seminar Series. *Academic Medicine* 71: 548–549.

Katz, D. A. 1999. Barriers between Guidelines and Improved Health Care: An Analysis of AHCPR's Unstable Angina Clinical Practice Guideline. *Health Services Research* 34: 377–389.

Katz, J. 1984. *The Silent World of Doctor and Patient*. New York: The Free Press.

Kaufman, S. R. 1993. *The Healer's Tale: Transforming Medicine and Culture*. Madison: University of Wisconsin Press.

Keating, P., and A. Cambrosio. 2000. Biomedical Platforms. *Configurations* 8(3): 337–387.

Kilgore, E. S. 1915. Clinical Records in Relation to Teaching and Research—A Plan to Promote Conservation and Utilization of Material. *Boston Medical and Surgical Journal* 173: 767–772.

Klazinga, N. S. 1997. *Quality Management of Medical Specialist Care in the Netherlands: An Explorative Study of its Nature and Development*. Overveen: Belvédère.

———. 1994. Compliance with Practice Guidelines: Clinical Autonomy Revisited. *Health Policy* 28: 51–66.

Knorr-Cetina, K. 1996. The Care of the Self and Blind Variation: The Disunity between Two Leading Sciences. In *The Disunity of Science: Boundaries, Contexts*, *and Power*, edited by P. Galison and D. J. Stump, 287–310. Stanford: Stanford University Press.

———. 1999. *Epistemic Cultures: How the Sciences Make Knowledge*. Cambridge, MA: Harvard University Press.

Korcok, M. 1994. Medical-Management Guidelines Being Developed with a Vengeance in US. *Canadian Medical Association Journal* 151: 1625–1627.

Kossoff, G., and W. L. Nyborg. 1989. Second World Federation of Ultrasound in Medicine and Biology Symposium on Safety and Standardization in Medical Ultrasound. *Ultrasound in Medicine and Biology* 15: 1–97.

Krantz, J. C. 1978. The Kefauver-Harris Amendment after Sixteen Years. *Military Medicine* 143: 883.

Krislov, S. 1997. *How Nations Choose Product Standards and Standards Change Nations*. Pittsburgh, PA: University of Pittsburgh Press.

Kurland, L. T., and C. A. Molgaard. 1981. The Patient Record in Epidemiology. *Scientific American* 245: 54–63.

Lachmund, J. 1998. Between Scrutiny and Treatment: Physical Diagnosis and the Restructuring of 19th Century Medical Practice. *Sociology of Health and Illness* 20: 779–801.

Laires, M. F., M. J. Ladeira, and J. P. Christensen, eds. 1995. *Health in the New Communications Age: Health Care Telematics for the 21st Century*. Amsterdam: IOS Press.

Lambert, B. L. 1996. Face and Politeness in Pharmacist-Physician Interaction. *Social Science and Medicine* 43: 1189–1198.

Latham, S. R. 2001. System and Responsibility: Three Readings of the IOM Report on Medical Error. *American Journal of Law and Medicine* 27: 163–179.

Latour, B. 1986. Visualisation and Cognition: Thinking with Eyes and Hands. *Knowledge and Society: Studies in the Sociology of Culture Past and Present* 6: 1–40.

———. 1987. *Science in Action: How to Follow Scientists and Engineers through Society*. Cambridge, MA: Harvard University Press.

———. 1992. Where are the Missing Massess? The Sociology of a Few Mundane Artefacts. In *Shaping Technology—Building Society: Studies in Sociotechnical Change*, edited by W. Bijker and J. Law, 225–258. Boston: MIT Press.

———. 1994. On Technical Mediation: Philosophy, Sociology, Genealogy. *Common Knowledge* 3: 29–64.

———. 1996. *Aramis, or the Love of Technology*. Cambridge, MA: Harvard University Press.

———. 1999. *Pandora's Hope: Essays on the Reality of Science Studies*. Cambridge, MA: Harvard University Press.

———. in press. Is There *Life* after Science Studies? A Novel Falsification Principle and Its Application to 'Body Talks'. *Body and Society*.

Law, J. 1987. Technology and Heterogeneous Engineering: The Case of Portuguese Expansion. In *The Social Construction of Technological Systems. New Directions in the Sociology and History of Technology*, edited by W. E. Bijker, T. P. Hughes, and T. J. Pinch, 111–134. Cambridge, MA: MIT Press.

Law, J., and J. Hassard, eds. 1999. *Actor Network Theory and After*. Oxford: Blackwell.

Lawrence, C. 1992. Democratic, Divine, and Heroic: The History and Historiography of Surgery. In *Medical Theory, Surgical Practice: Studies in the History of Surgery*, edited by C. Lawrence, 1–47. London: Routledge.

Lee, N., and S. Brown. 1994. Otherness and the Actor-Network: The Undiscovered Continent. *American Behavioral Scientist* 37: 772–790.

Levine, M. R. 1987. *A Physician's Guide to Utilization Review*. Philadelphia: F. A. Davis Company.

Lewinski-Corwin, E. H. 1922. Medical Case Recording in Hospitals. *Journal of the American Medical Association* 78: 604–605.

Lewis, R. 2001. The Return of Thalidomide. *The Scientist* 15: 1–14.

Liang, M. H. 1992. From America: Cookbook Medicine and Food for Thought: Practice Guideline Development in the USA. *Annals of Rheumatic Diseases* 51: 1257–1258.

Light, D. 1979. Uncertainty and Control in Professional Training. *Journal of Health and Social Behavior* 20: 310–322.

———. 1993. Countervailing Power: The Changing Character of the Medical Profession in the United States. In *The Changing Medical Profession: An International Perspective*, edited by F. W. Hafferty and J. B. McKinlay, 69–80. New York: Oxford University Press.

———. 2000. The Medical Profession and Organizational Change: From Professional Dominance to Countervailing Power. In *Handbook of Medical Sociology*, edited by C. E. Bird, P. Conrad, and A. M. Fremont, 201–217. Upper Saddle River, NJ: Prentice-Hall.

Light, D., and D. Hughes. 2001. A Sociological Perspective on Rationing: Power, Rhetoric, and Situated Practices. *Sociology of Health and Illness* 23: 551–569.

Light, D. W., and S. Levine. 1988. The Changing Character of the Medical Profession: A Theoretical Overview. *The Milbank Quarterly* 66: 10–32.

LISV. 1997. *Interne evaluatie standaarden*. Amsterdam: LISV.

Lohr, K. N., K. Eleazer, and J. Mauskopf. 1998. Health Policy Issues and Applications of Evidence-Based Medicine and Clinical Practice Guidelines. *Health Policy* 46: 1–9.

Long, D. E., and J. Golden. 1989. *The American General Hospital*. Ithaca and London: Cornell University Press.

Löwy, I. 1997. *Between Bench and Bedside: Science, Healing and Interleukin-2 in a Cancer Ward*. Cambridge, MA: Harvard University Press.

Lundberg, N., and O. Hanseth. 2001. Standardization Strategies in Practice—Examples from Health Care. In *Strategies for Healthcare Information Systems*, edited by R. Stegwee and T. Spil, 46–65. Hershey: Idea Group Publishing.

Lynaugh, J. E. 1989. From Respectable Domesticity to Medical Efficiency: The Changing Kansas City Hospital, 1875–1920. In *The American General Hospital*, edited by D. E. Long and J. L. Golden, 21–39. Ithaca and London: Cornell University Press.

Lynch, M. 1993. *Scientific Practice and Ordinary Action: Ethnomethodology and So-cial Studies of Science*. New York: Cambridge University Press.

Mann, R. D. 1987. *Adverse Drug Reactions: The Scale and Nature of the Problem and the Way Forward*. Camforth, UK: Parthenon.

Manning, N. 2002. Actor Networks, Policy Networks and Personality Disorder. *Sociology of Health and Illness* 24: 644–666.

Mannix, J. R. 1935. Medical Records—Are They Worth the Price? *Modern Hospital* 45: 71–72.

Mansholt, W. H. 1931. Wat kunnen Europeesche en Amerikaansche zieken-huizen werderkeerig van elkaar leeren. *Het Ziekenhuiswezen* 4: 28–42.

Marshall, T. 1997. Scientific Knowledge in Medicine: A New Clinical Epistemol-ogy. *Journal of Evaluation in Clinical Practice* 3: 133–138.

Martin, E. 1987. *The Woman in the Body: A Cultural Analysis of Reproduction*. Boston, MA: Beacon Press.

Massaro, T. A. 1993. Introducing Physician Order Entry at a Major Academic Medical Center: I. Impact on Organizational Culture and Behavior. *Academic Medicine* 68: 20–25.

Matthews, J. R. 1995. *Quantification and the Quest for Medical Certainty*. Princeton: Princeton University Press.

————. 1999. Practice Guidelines and Tort Reform: The Legal System Con-fronts the Technocratic Wish. *Journal of Health Politics, Policy and Law* 24: 275–304.

May, W. E. 1985. Consensus or Coercion. *Journal of the American Medical Associ-ation* 254: 1077.

McCloskey, J., and G. Bulechek. 2000. *Nursing Interventions Classification (NIC)*. St. Louis: Mosby-Year Book.

McDonald, C. J., S. L. Hui, D. M. Smith, W. M. Tierney, S. J. Cohen, M. Wein-berger, and G. P. McGabe. 1984. Reminders to Physicians from an Introspec-tive Computer Medical Record: A Two-Year Randomized Trial. *Annals of In-ternal Medicine* 100: 130–138.

McGlynn, E. A. 1998. The Outcomes Utility Index: Will Outcomes Data Tell Us What We Want to Know? *International Journal of Quality Health Care* 10: 485–490.

McIntyre, K. 2001. Medicolegal Implications of the Consensus Conference. *Chest* 119: S337–S343.

Meershoek, A. 1999. *Weer aan het werk. Verzekeringsgeneeskundige verzuimbegeleid-ing als onderhandeling over verantwoordelijkheden*. Maastricht: Proefschrift Uni-versiteit Maastricht.

Merritt, A. T., D. Palmer, D. A. Bergman, and P. H. Shiono. 1997. Clinical Practice Guidelines in Pediatric and Newborn Medicine: Implications for Their Use in Practice. *Pediatrics* 99: 100–114.

Merton, R., G. G. Reader, and P. L. Kendall. 1957. *The Student-Physician: Intro-ductory Studies in the Sociology of Medical Education*. Cambridge, MA: Harvard University Press for the Commonwealth Fund.

Miles, A., P. Bentley, A. Polychronis, and J. Grey. 1997. Evidence-Based Medicine: Why All the Fuss? This is Why. *Journal of Evaluation in Clinical Practice* 3: 83–86.

Millenson, M. L. 1997. *Demanding Medical Excellence. Doctors and Accountability in the Information Age.* Chicago: University of Chicago Press.

Miller, L. W., S. H. Kubo, J. B. Young, L. W. Stevenson, L. Evan, and M. R. Constanzo. 1995. Report of the Consensus Conference on Candidate Selection for Heart Transplantation. *Journal of Heart and Lung Transplant* 14: 562–571.

Mintzberg, H. 1979. *The Structuring of Organizations.* Englewood Cliffs: Prentice-Hall.

Mitchell, J. P. 2000. Guideline Implementation in the Department of Defense. *Chest* 118: S65–S69.

Mol, A., and J. Law. 1994. Regions, Networks and Fluids: Anaemia and Social Topology. *Social Studies of Science* 24: 641–671.

Mol, A., and P. van Lieshout. 1989. *Ziek is het woord niet. Medicalisering, normalisering en de veranderende taal van huisartsgeneeskunde en geestelijke gezondheidszorg, 1945–1985.* Nijmegen: SUN.

Morgan, E. T., ed. 1989. *Efficiency, Scientific Management and Hospital Standardization.* New York and London: Garland Publishing.

Morris, J. 1991. *Pride Against Prejudice: Transforming Attitudes to Disability.* London: The Women's Press.

Mulrow, C. D. 1994. Rationale for Systematic Reviews. *British Medical Journal* 309: 597–599.

Munger, C. W. 1928. Hospital Case Records and Professional Standing Orders. *Modern Hospital* 30: 99–106.

Noble, D. F. 1984. *Forces of Production: A Social History of Industrial Automation.* Oxford and New York: Oxford University Press.

Nony, P., M. Cucherat, and J.-P. Boissel. 1999. Implication of Evidence-Based Medicine in Prescription Guidelines Taught to French Medical Students: Current Status in the Cardiovascular Field. *Clinical Pharmacology and Therapeutics* 66: 173–184.

Norman, G. R., and S. I. Shannon. 1998. Effectiveness of Instruction in Critical Appraisal (Evidence-Based Medicine) Skills: A Critical Appraisal. *Canadian Medical Association Journal* 158: 177–181.

Nortington Gamble, V. 1989. The Negro Hospital Renaissance: The Black Hospital Movement, 1920–1945. In *The American General Hospital,* edited by D. E. Long and J. Golden, 82–105. Ithaca and London: Cornell University Press.

O'Connell, J. 1993. Metrology: The Creation of Universality by the Circulation of Particulars. *Social Studies of Science* 23: 129–173.

Olsen, R. T. 1920. Keeping Records at Englewood Hospital, Chicago. *Modern Hospital* 15: 269–271.

Ornstein, S. M., R. B. Oates, and G. N. Fox. 1992. The Computer-Based Medical Record: Current Status. *Journal of Family Practice* 35(5): 347–362.

Paauw, D. S. 1999. Did We Learn Evidence-Based Medicine in Medical School? Some Common Medical Mythology. *Journal of the American Board of Family Practice* 12(2): 143–150.

Pasveer, B. 1989. Knowledge of Shadows: The Introduction of X-ray Images in Medicine. *Sociology of Health and Illness* 11: 360–381.

———. 1992. *Shadows of Knowledge. Making a Representing Practice in Medicine: X-ray Pictures and Pulmonary Tuberculosis, 1895–1930.* Universiteit van Amsterdam.

Patrias, K., R. L. Gordner, and S. Groft. 1997. *Thalidomide: Potential Benefits and Risks.* Bethesda, MD: National Library of Medicine.

Pearl, R. 1921. Modern Methods in Handling Hospital Statistics. *Johns Hopkins Hospital Bulletin* 32: 184–194.

Pearson, S. D. C. Z. Margolis, S. Davis, L. K. Schreier, and L. K. Gottlieb. 1992. The Clinical Algorithm Nosology: A Method for Comparing Algorithmic Guidelines. *Medical Decision Making* 12: 123–131.

Pellegrino, E. D. 1996. The Autopsy: Some Ethical Reflections on the Obligations of Pathologists, Hospitals, Families and Society. *Archives of Pathology and Laboratory Medicine* 120: 739–742.

Perrow, C. 1984. *Normal Accidents: Living with High Risk Technologies.* New York: Basic Books.

Phipps, P. A. 1990. Industrial and Occupational Change in Pharmacy: Prescription for Feminization. In *Job Queues, Gender Queues: Explaining Women's Inroads into Male Occupations,* edited by B. F. Reskin and P. A. Roos, 111–128. Philadelphia: Temple University Press.

Pinch, T. T., and W. E. Bijker. 1984. The Social Construction of Facts and Artefacts: Or How the Sociology of Science and the Sociology of Technology Might Benefit Each Other. *Social Studies of Science* 14: 399–441.

Porter, R. 1997. *The Greatest Benefit to Mankind: A Medical History of Humanity.* New York: W. W. Norton and Company.

Porter, T. M. 1995. *Trust in Numbers: Objectivity in Science and Public Life.* Princeton: Princeton University Press.

Rapp, R. 1998. Refusing Prenatal Diagnosis: The Meanings of Bioscience in a Multicultural World. *Science, Technology, and Human Values* 23: 45–71.

Rappolt, S. M. 1997. Clinical Guidelines and the Fate of Medical Autonomy in Ontario. *Social Science and Medicine* 44: 977–987.

Reiser, S. J. 1978. *Medicine and the Reign of Technology.* Cambridge: Cambridge University Press.

———. 1984. Creating Form Out of Mass: The Development of the Medical Record. In *Transformation and Tradition in the Sciences: Essays in Honor of I. Bernard Cohen,* edited by E. Mendelsohn, 303–316. New York: Cambridge University Press.

———. 1991a. The Clinical Record in Medicine. Part 1: Learning from Cases. *Annals of Internal Medicine* 114: 902–907.

———. 1991b. The Clinical Record in Medicine. Part 2: Reforming Content and Purpose. *Annals of Internal Medicine* 114: 980–985.

Relman, A. S. 1980. The New Medical-Industrial Complex. *New England Journal of Medicine* 303: 963–970.

Reverby, S. 1981. Stealing the Golden Eggs: Ernest Amory Codman and the Science and Management of Medicine. *Bulletin of the History of Medicine* 55: 156–271.

Rhew, D. C., D. C. Riedinger, M. Sandhu, C. Bowers, N. Greenold, and S. R. Weingarten. 1998. A Prospective, Multicenter Study of a Pneumonia Practice Guideline. *Chest* 114: 115–119.

Richard, E. 1991. *Vitamin C and Cancer: Medicine or Politics*. London: Macmillan.

Ritzer, G. 1992. *The McDonaldization of Society: An Investigation into the Changing Character of Contemporary Social Life*. Thousand Oaks, CA: Pine Forge.

Ritzer, G., and D. Walczak. 1988. Rationalization and the Deprofessionalization of Physicians. *Social Forces* 67: 1–22.

Rodwin, M. A. 2001. The Politics of Evidence-Based Medicine. *Journal of Health Politics, Policy and Law* 26: 439–446.

Rogers, Y. 1993. Coordinating Computer-Mediated Work. *Computer Supported Cooperative Work* 1: 295–315.

Rolnick, S. J., Flores, S. K., O'Fallon, A. M., and N. R. Vanderburg. 2000. The Implementation of Clinical Guidelines in a Managed Care Setting: Implications for Children with Special Health Care Needs. *Managed Care Quarterly* 8: 29–38.

Rosenberg, C. E. 1987. *The Care of Strangers: The Rise of America's Hospital System*. New York: Basic Books.

Rosoff, A. J. 2001. Evidence-Based Medicine and the Law: The Courts Confront Clinical Practice Guidelines. *Journal of Health Politics, Policy and Law* 26: 327–368.

Rosser, W. W., D. Davis, and E. Gilbart. 2001. Assessing Guidelines for Use in Family Practice. *Journal of Family Practice* 50: 974–975.

Rothman, D. J. 1991. *Strangers at the Bedside: A History of How Law and Bioethics Transformed Medical Decision Making*. New York: Basic Books.

Sackett, D. L., B. R. Haynes, and P. Tugwell. 1985. *Clinical Epidemiology: A Basic Science for Clinical Medicine*. Boston: Little, Brown.

Sackett, D. L., and W. M. C. Rosenberg. 1995. The Need for Evidence-Based Medicine. *Journal of the Royal Society of Medicine* 88: 620–624.

Sackett, D. L., W. M. C. Rosenberg, J. A. Gray, B. R. Haynes, and W. S. Richardson. 1996. Evidence Based Medicine: What It Is and What It Isn't. *British Medical Journal* 312: 71–72.

Sackett, D. L., S. E. Straus, W. S. Richardson, W. Rosenberg, and B. R. Haynes. 2000. *Evidence-Based Medicine: How to Practice and Teach EBM*. Edinburgh: Churchill Livingstone.

Sanders, A. B. 1999. Do We Need a Clinical Decision Rule for the Discontinuation of Cardiac Arrest Resuscitations? *Archives of Internal Medicine* 159: 119–121.

Santucci, G., J. O. Asbjoern, E. F. Bach, B. Barber, J. H. von Bemmel, D. Bravak, W. von Emmeken, and C. Greinacher. 1990. Rationale for a Community Strategy in the Field of Information and Communications Technologies Applied to Health Care. *Methods of Information in Medicine* 29: 84–91.

Saver, B. G. 1996. Whose Guideline is it Anyway? *Archives of Family Medicine* 5: 532–534.

Savoie, I., Kazanjian, A., and K. Bassett. 2000. Do Clinical Practice Guidelines Reflect Research Evidence? *Journal of Health Services Research and Policy* 5: 76–82.

Scally, G., and L. J. Donaldson. 1998. The NHS's 50 Anniversary: Clinical Governance and the Drive for Quality Improvement in the New NHS in England. *British Medical Journal* 317: 61–65.

Schlesinger, J. M., H. G. Bradford, and K. M. Perreira. 1997. Medical Professionalism Under Managed Care: The Pros and Cons of Utilization Review. *Health Affairs* 16: 105–124.

Schmidt, K., and L. Bannon. 1992. Taking CSCW Seriously: Supporting Articulation Work. *Computer Supported Cooperative Work* 1: 7–40.

Schmidt, K., and C. Simone. 1996. Coordination Mechanisms: Towards a Conceptual Foundation of CSCW Systems Design. *Computer Supported Cooperative Work* 5: 155–200.

Schmidt, S. K., and R. Werle. 1998. *Coordinating Technology: Studies in the International Standardization of Telecommunications*. Cambridge, MA: MIT Press.

Schoute, D. 1925. Stafvorming in Amerikaansche en in Nederlandsche ziekenhuizen. *Het Ziekenhuis* 16: 106–113.

Secretary of State for Health. 1997. *The New NHS*. London: Stationary Office.

Shapin, S. 1989. The Invisible Technician. *American Scientist* 77: 554–563.

Shapin, S., and S. Schaffer. 1985. *Leviathan and the Air-Pump: Hobbes, Boyle, and the Experimental Life*. Princeton: Princeton University Press.

Shapiro, S. 1997. Degrees of Freedom: The Interaction of Standards of Practice and Engineering Judgment. *Science, Technology and Human Values* 22: 286–316.

Shear, M. K., and J. D. Maser. 1994. Standardized Assessment for Panic Disorder Research. *Archives of General Psychiatry* 51: 346–354.

Shenhav, Y. 1999. *Manufacturing Rationality*. Oxford: Oxford University Press.

Siberry, G. K., and R. Iannone, eds. 2000. *The Harriet Lane Handbook: A Manual for Pediatric House Officers*. St. Louis: Mosby.

Silverman, D. 1987. *Communication in Medical Practice*. London: Sage.

Singleton, V. 1998. Stabilizing Instabilities: The Laboratory in the UK Cervical Screening Program. In *Differences in Medicine: Unraveling Practices, Techniques and Bodies*, edited by M. Berg and A. Mol, 86–104. Durham: Duke University Press.

Sitkin, S. B., and K. M. Sutcliffe. 1991. Dispensing Legitimacy: The Influence of Professional, Organizational, and Legal Controls on Pharmacist Behavior. *Research in the Sociology of Organizations* 8: 269–295.

Slobe, F. W. 1923. Applying Minimal Standards to Hospitals. *Modern Hospital* 20: 166–168.

Smart, S., and C. Williams. 1997. Evidence-Based Advertising? Half of Drug Advertisements in BMJ over Six Months Cited No Supportive Evidence. *British Medical Journal* 1622–1623.

Smith, D. 1978. "K Is Mentally Ill": The Anatomy of a Factual Account. *Sociology* 12: 23–53.

———. 1990. *Texts, Facts, and Femininity: Exploring the Relations of Ruling.* London: Routledge.

Smith, D. W. H. 1913. Discussion on "The statistical experience data of the Johns Hopkins Hosspital, 1892–1911." *Johns Hopkins Hospital Bulletin* 226–227.

Smith, W. R. 2000. Evidence for the Effectiveness of Techniques to Change Physician Behavior. *Chest* 118: S8–S17.

Solberg, L. I. 2000. Guideline Implementation: What the Literature Doesn't Tell Us. *Joint Commission Journal on Quality Improvement* 26: 525–537.

Sonnad, S. S., and S. E. Foreman. 1997. An Incentive Approach to Physician Implementation of Medical Practice Guidelines. *Health Economics* 6: 467–477.

Sox , J. H. C., and S. Woloshin. 2000. How Many Deaths are due to Medical Error? Getting the Number Right. *Effects of Clinical Practice* 3: 277–283.

Star, S. L. 1991. The Sociology of the Invisible: The Primacy of Work in the Writings of Anselm Strauss. In *Social Organization and Social Process: Essays in Honor of Anselm Strauss,* edited by D. R. Maines, 265–283. Hawthorne: Aldine de Gruyter.

Star, S. L., and J. R. Griesemer. 1989. Institutional Ecology, "Translations," and Boundary Objects: Amateurs and Professionals in Berkely's Museum of Vertebrate Zoology, 1907–39. *Social Studies of Science* 19: 387–420.

Star, S. L., and K. Ruhleder. 1996. Steps towards an Ecology of Infrastructure: Design and Access for Large Information Spaces. *Information Systems Research* 7: 111.

Star, S. L., and A. Strauss. 1999. Layers of Silence, Arenas of Voice: The Ecology Visible and Invisible Work. *Computer Supported Cooperative Work* 8(12): 9–31.

Starr, P. 1982. *The Social Transformation of American Medicine.* New York: Basic Books.

Stengers, I. 1997. *Power and Invention: Situating Science.* Minneapolis: University of Minnesota Press.

Stevens, H. P. 1919. Case Records and Histories in the Smaller Hospitals. *Boston Medical and Surgical Journal* 181: 324–329.

Stevens, R. 1989. *In Sickness and in Wealth: American Hospitals in the Twentieth Century.* New York: Basic Books.

Stokes, J. H., R. A. Kern, and L. K. Ferguson. 1933. What Sixty-Six Hospitals Think of the Central Unit Record System. *Modern Hospital* 40: 87–92.

Strading, J. R., and R. J. O. Davies. 1997. The Unacceptable Face of Evidence-Based Medicine. *Journal of Evaluation in Clinical Practice* 3: 99–103.

Strauss, A. 1987. *Qualitative Analysis for Social Scientists.* Cambridge: Cambridge University Press.

Strumwasser, I., N. V. Paranjpe, D. L. Ronis, D. Share, and L. J. Sell. 1990. Reliability and Validity of Utilization Review Criteria: Appropriateness Evaluation Protocol, Standardized Medreview Instrument, and Intensity-Severity-Discharge Criteria. *Medical Care* 28: 95–109.

Suchman, L. 1987. *Plans and Situated Actions: The Problem of Human-Machine Communication.* Cambridge: Cambridge University Press.

————. 1993. Technologies of Accountability: Of Lizards and Aeroplanes. In *Technology in Working Order: Studies of Work, Interaction, and Technology,* edited by G. Button, 113–126. London: Routledge.

Sunday Times Insight Team. 1979. *Suffer the Children: The Story of Thalidomide.* London: Andre Deutch.

Tallon, D., J. Chard, and P. Dieppe. 2000. Relation between Agendas of the Research Community and the Research Consumer. *Lancet* 2037–2040.

Tanenbaum, S. J. 1994. Knowing and Acting in Medical Practice: The Epistemological Politics of Outcomes Research. *Journal of Health Politics, Policy and Law* 19: 27–44.

Taylor, F. W. 1914. *The Principles of Scientific Management.* New York and London: Harper and Brothers Publishers.

Timmermans, S. 1999a. Mutual Tuning of Multiple Trajectories. *Symbolic Interaction* 21: 225–240.

————. 1999b. *Sudden Death and the Myth of CPR.* Philadelphia: Temple University Press.

Timmermans, S., G. C. Bowker, and L. S. Star. 1998. The Architecture of Difference: Visibility, Control, and Comparability in Building a Nursing Interventions Classification. In *Differences in Medicine,* edited by M. Berg and A. Mol, 202–225. Durham: Duke University Press.

Tunis, S., S. R. Hayward, M. C. Wilson, M. R. Rubin, E. B. Bass, M. Johnston, and E. P. Steinberg. 1994a. Internists' Attitudes about Clinical Practice Guidelines. *Annals of Internal Medicine* 120: 956–963.

Turnberg, L. 1997. *Biological Standardization and Control: The Scientific Basis of Standardization and Quality Control/Safety Monitoring of Biological Substances Used in Medicine.* Geneva: World Health Organization.

U.S. Preventive Services Task Force. 1996. *Guide to Clinical Preventive Services.* Baltimore: Williams and Wilkins.

Vakil, N. B. 2001. Evidence-Based Health Care: Making Health Policy and Management Decisions. *Managed Care* 10: 22–24.

van der Lei, J., E. van der Does, A. J. Man in 't Veld, M. A. Musen, and J. H. van Bemmel. 1993. Response of General Practitioners to Computer-Generated Critiques of Hypertension Therapy. *Methods of Information in Medicine* 32: 146–153.

Vaughan, D. 1996. *The Challenger Launch Decision: Risky Technology, Culture and Deviance at NASA.* Chicago: University of Chicago Press.

Vogel, D. 1990. When Consumers Oppose Consumer Protection: The Politics of Regulatory Backlash. *Journal of Public Policy* 10(4): 449–470.

Vogel, M. J., and C. E. Rosenberg, ed. 1979. *The Therapeutic Revolution: Essays in the Social History of American Medicine*. Philadelphia: University of Pennsylvania Press.

Warner, J. H. 1985. Science in Medicine. *Osiris* 1 (2nd series): 37–58.

———. 1986. *The Therapeutic Perspective: Medical Practice, Knowledge and Identity in America, 1820–1885*. Cambridge, MA: Harvard University Press.

Weed, L. L. 1985. The Computer as a New Basis for Analytical Clinical Practice: Coupling Individual Problems with Medical Knowledge. *Mount Sinai Journal of Medicine* 52: 94–98.

Weingarten, S. 2000. Translating Practice Guidelines into Patient Care. *Chest* 118: S4–S7.

Weiss, K. B., and R. Wagner. 2000. Performance Measurement Through Audit, Feedback, and Profiling as Tools for Improving Clinical Care. *Chest* 118: S53–S58.

Welch, G. H., and J. D. Lurie. 2000. Teaching Evidence-Based Medicine: Caveats and Challenges. *Academic Medicine* 75: 235–240.

Welsh, J. 1995. Banned in U.S. for Causing Birth Defects, Thalidomide Returns as an AIDS Drug. *Wall Street Journal*.

Wennberg, J. E. 1984. Dealing with Medical Practice Variation: A Proposal for Action. *Health Affairs* 3: 6–32.

———. 1999. *The Dartmouth Atlas of Health Care 1999*. Chicago: American Hospital Publishing.

Whiting Myers, G. 1932. How the Record Librarian Serves Three Masters Impartially. *Modern Hospital* 39: 64–66.

Wiener, C. L. 2000. *The Elusive Quest: Accountability in Hospitals*. New York: Aldine de Gruyter.

Wilkinson, B. 1983. *The Shopfloor Politics of New Technology*. London: Heinemann Educational Books.

Williamson, C. 1992. *Whose Standards? Consumer and Professional Standards in Health Care*. Buckingham and Philadelphia: Open University Press.

Winthereik, B. R. In press. Achieving Localization in an Information System for Primary Care: Codes, Classifications and Accuracy. *Methods of Information in Medicine*.

Wise, N. M., ed. 1995. *The Values of Precision*. Princeton: Princeton University Press.

Wolff, N., and M. Schlesinger. 1998. Risk, Motives, and Styles of Utilization Review: A Cross-Condition Comparison. *Social Science and Medicine* 47: 911–926.

Woolf, S. H., C. G. DiGiuseppi, D. Atkins, and D. B. Kamerow. 1996. Developing Evidence-Based Clinical Practice Guidelines. *Annual Review of Public Health* 17: 511–538.

Woolf, S. H., R. Grol, A. Hutchinson, M. Eccles, and J. Grimshaw. 1999. Potential Benefits, Limitations, and Harms of Clinical Guidelines. *British Medical Journal* 318: 527–530.

Wynia, M. K. 1997. Economic Analyses, the Medical Commons, and Patients' Dilemmas: What is the Physician's Role? *Journal of Investigative Medicine* 45: 35–43.

Yates, J. 1989. *Control through Communication: The Rise of System in American Management*. Baltimore: Johns Hopkins University Press.

Zinberg, S. 1998. Practice Guidelines—A Continuing Debate. *Clinical Obstetrics and Gynecology* 41: 343–347.

Zuboff, S. 1988. *In the Age of the Smart Machine. The Future of Work and Power*. New York: Basic Books.

Index

Abbott, Andrew, 84, 85
ACP Journal Club, The, 5
actor-network theory, 22, 221n. 42, 224–225n. 26
adult learning theory, 146
Alder, Ken, 229n. 51
American Academy of Pediatrics, 111, 149
American Association of Health Plans, 7
American Association of Medical Colleges, 142
American College of Gynecologists and Obstetricians, 86–87, 104, 105, 111
American College of Physicians, 84
American College of Surgeons (ACS), 10, 32, 35–38, 198
American Heart Association, 3, 69; and CPR protocols, 82
American Hospital Association, 220n. 34
American Medical Association (AMA), 7; opposition to adoption of clinical practice guidelines as a legal standard, 110; reform of medical education, 35
American Pharmaceutical Association, 186
American Psychiatric Association, 111
American Railway Association, 9
Annals of Internal Medicine, 5
Appropriateness Evaluation Protocol (AEP), 102
Archives of Internal Medicine, 83
Armstrong, David, 97
Aronowitz, R. A., 27
Atkinson, P., 151, 152, 154, 158, 234n. 31
autonomy, 114–115; clinical autonomy, 84, 87, 88, 90, 98; professional autonomy, 84, 87, 227n. 11; and utilization review firms, 103–104. *See also* clinical practice guidelines

Bandolier, 5
Beck, Ulrich, 169
Belkin, Gary, 107
Bell, Susan, 235n. 25
benchmarking, 105
Berwick, Donald, 205
Best Evidence, 5
Best Evidence database, 152
Bosk, Charles, 159
Bottomley, J. T., 53
Bowker, Geof, 192
Brandeis, Louis, 11
British Medical Journal, 5, 97–98

Canadian Thalidomide Victims Association, 184
cardiopulmonary resuscitation (CPR), 1–2, 82–83
carepath, 224n. 6
Carville leprosy treatment center, 172, 173, 179, 181, 236n. 48
Celgene, 166, 167, 173–176, 188–189. *See also* S.T.E.P.S. program
Challenger launch decision, 168
clinical epidemiology, 15
clinical pathway, 224n. 6
clinical practice guidelines, 3, 26, 82–86; in Canada, 105–106; and compliance, 95–96; definition of, 3; and the distribution of risk, 167–169; and emerging professions, 90–94; and established professions, 86–90; and external regulation, 99–101; and Freidson's "market shelter," 85, 94, 104, 107; guideline formulation, 95–96; guideline implementation, 95–96; "guidelines for clinical guidelines," 95–96; lack of awareness of, 94–95; and the law, 108–112; and noncompliance, 96–98, 101; and objectivity, 117–119; overload

265